DISEASES & DISORDERS

Sickle Cell Disease

Lizabeth Peak

LUCENT BOOKS
A part of Gale, Cengage Learning

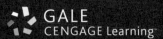
GALE
CENGAGE Learning

Detroit • New York • San Francisco • New Haven, Conn • Waterville, Maine • London

616.1

Pea

3/14

GALE
CENGAGE Learning·

© 2008 Gale, a part of Cengage Learning

For more information, contact
Lucent Books
27500 Drake Rd.
Farmington Hills, MI 48331-3535
Or you can visit our Internet site at gale.cengage.com

LIBRARY OF CONGRESS CATALOGING-IN-PUBLICATION DATA

Peak, Lizabeth.
  Sickle Cell Disease / by Lizabeth Peak.
     p. cm. — (Diseases and disorders)
  Includes bibliographical references and index.
  ISBN 978-1-59018-864-4 (hardcover)
  1. Sickle cell anemia—Popular works. I. Title.
  RC641.7.S5P43 2008
  616.1'527—dc22

                                                                     2007030613

ISBN-10: 1-59018-864-0

Printed in the United States of America
   3 4 5 6 7 12 11 10 09 08

Table of Contents

"The Most Difficult Puzzles Ever Devised"

Charles Best, one of the pioneers in the search for a cure for diabetes, once explained what it is about medical research that intrigued him so. "It's not just the gratification of knowing one is helping people," he confided, "although that probably is a more heroic and selfless motivation. Those feelings may enter in, but truly, what I find best is the feeling of going toe to toe with nature, of trying to solve the most difficult puzzles ever devised. The answers are there somewhere, those keys that will solve the puzzle and make the patient well. But how will those keys be found?"

Since the dawn of civilization, nothing has so puzzled people—and often frightened them, as well—as the onset of illness in a body or mind that had seemed healthy before. A seizure, the inability of a heart to pump, the sudden deterioration of muscle tone in a small child—being unable to reverse such conditions or even to understand why they occur was unspeakably frustrating to healers. Even before there were names for such conditions, even before they were understood at all, each was a reminder of how complex the human body was, and how vulnerable.

While our grappling with understanding diseases has been frustrating at times, it has also provided some of humankind's most heroic accomplishments. Alexander Fleming's accidental discovery in 1928 of a mold that could be turned into penicillin has resulted in the saving of untold millions of lives. The isolation of the enzyme insulin has reversed what was once a death sentence for anyone with diabetes. There have been great strides in combating conditions for which there is not yet a cure, too. Medicines can help AIDS patients live longer, diagnostic tools such as mammography and ultrasounds can help doctors find tumors while they are treatable, and laser surgery techniques have made the most intricate, minute operations routine.

This "toe-to-toe" competition with diseases and disorders is even more remarkable when seen in a historical continuum. An astonishing amount of progress has been made in a very short time. Just two hundred years ago, the existence of germs as a cause of some diseases was unknown. In fact, it was less than 150 years ago that a British surgeon named Joseph Lister had difficulty persuading his fellow doctors that washing their hands before delivering a baby might increase the chances of a healthy delivery (especially if they had just attended to a diseased patient)!

Each book in Lucent's Diseases and Disorders series explores a disease or disorder and the knowledge that has been accumulated (or discarded) by doctors through the years. Each book also examines the tools used for pinpointing a diagnosis, as well as the various means that are used to treat or cure a disease. Finally, new ideas are presented—techniques or medicines that may be on the horizon.

Frustration and disappointment are still part of medicine, for not every disease or condition can be cured or prevented. But the limitations of knowledge are being pushed outward constantly; the "most difficult puzzles ever devised" are finding challengers every day.

An Old Disease with a New Name

In 1846, a runaway slave was executed for the murder of another runaway slave. One hour after the hanging, the court allowed the unclaimed body to be "delivered to any surgeon who demanded it." It fell into the hands of one Dr. R. Lebby, who performed an autopsy. In his report, Dr. Lebby noted the slave's unusual build, certain symptoms he had suffered during his life, and "the strange phenomenon of a man having lived without a spleen."[1] The findings were typical of a person suffering from the blood disease now called sickle cell disease, but Dr. Lebby could not have known this because the disease had not yet been identified. Although the disease was taking the lives of thousands of people every year, it had no name and no treatment.

The first formal description of sickle cell disease came about fifty years later, when, in 1910, cardiologist Dr. James Herrick of Chicago reported "peculiar elongated and sickle-shaped" red blood cells in "an intelligent Negro of twenty,"[2] a college student named Walter Clement Noel from the Caribbean island of Grenada. Six years earlier, Walter had come to Dr. Herrick because of shortness of breath, pain in his abdomen and in his muscles, headaches, dizziness, and skin ulcers on his legs. When Dr. Ernest Irons, an intern at the hospital, examined a sample of Walter's blood under a microscope, he noticed elongated, abnormally curved red cells in the blood and drew sketches of them. Dr. Herrick spent the

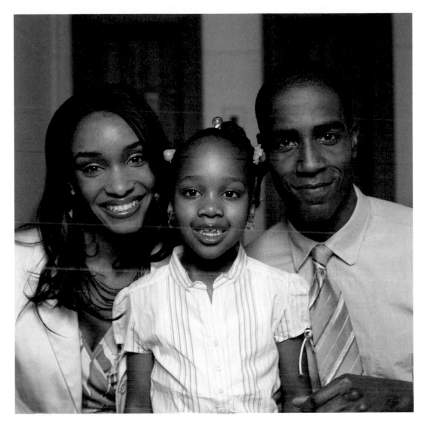

Although sickle cell disease can affect anyone, it most commonly appears in African Americans.

next six years studying Walter's disease and devising treatments for the symptoms. His 1910 report was the first medical report ever published about the strange disease. Other doctors began to pay more attention to their patients who had similar symptoms, and a pattern was soon discovered. After more cases were discovered and described, the disease was given the name "sickle cell anemia."

Sickle Cell Disease Today

Today, sickle cell disease is the most common genetic disease in the United States. Sickle cell can affect anyone of any race or nationality, but because it is an inherited disorder, passed from parent to child, it tends to appear mostly in certain ethnic groups. It affects over seventy thousand people in the United States, most commonly African Americans, with millions more affected around the world. Besides those of African descent, it also tends to appear in people of Hispanic, Turkish, Arabian, Greek, Indian, and Italian ancestry. It occurs in about one in every five hundred African American births and one in every one thousand to fourteen hundred Hispanic American births. According to the Sickle Cell Disease Association of America (SCDAA), sickle cell is responsible for approximately seven hundred fifty thousand hospitalizations every year, at a cost of about $475 million annually.

Thanks to improved understanding of the nature of the disease, which has led to earlier detection and better treatment, the quality of life and the life expectancy for patients with sickle cell disease has increased tremendously over the last thirty years. Treatment of the long-term complications of the disease has also improved. According to a study done in 1973, the average life expectancy for someone with Sickle Cell was only about fourteen years. By 1993, it had improved to forty-two years for men and forty-eight years for women. For people with a milder form of the disease, called sickle cell-hemoglobin C, the average life span extends into the sixties for both sexes.

Knowledge Is Power

Sickle cell disease is a very serious disorder with many symptoms and potentially life-threatening complications. Complications such as stroke can be severe and can occur very suddenly. Management of the symptoms can be quite complicated. For these reasons, it is critical for sickle cell patients and their families to be thoroughly knowledgeable about this disease. They must be able to follow the doctor's instructions and have a clear understanding of the reasons for those instructions. They also need to understand the role of medications, especially pain medications. Friends, teachers, other caregivers, and employers also need to be aware of the special health needs of the person with sickle cell disease. They must be able to recognize the signs of a painful sickle cell crisis and know what to do so that the pain can be treated promptly. All those who are involved in the person's life must be able to recognize the signs of possible complications, such as stroke, and be prepared to quickly get the help the person needs.

Patients, families, and friends also need to learn how to cope with the potentially overwhelming stress and emotional strain this disease can cause. Children and teens who have sickle cell often feel very different and set apart from their peers because of all the special needs they have. As one teenage girl with sickle cell explains:

> For as long as I can remember I have longed to be normal, and sometimes that longing made my life even harder than it was already. I was ashamed to be ill, and sometimes angry that pain episodes and other medical problems kept me from living what seemed to be the free and easy lives of my friends.[3]

In addition to the patient's doctor, organizations such as the SCDAA, the March of Dimes, and the American Sickle Cell Anemia Association, as well as many books and Web sites, offer support and information about the disease. Local support groups exist in most communities, offering financial, emotional, and psychological support. Although research funding is still relatively low compared to other diseases such as cancer and heart disease, progress is being made every day, bringing us closer to a safe and effective cure for sickle cell disease.

CHAPTER ONE

What Is Sickle Cell Disease?

Eli Hill had been enrolled in school for only two weeks when his teacher called his home, frantic. His mother, Deb, raced to the school to find Eli on the floor, his teacher supporting his head. "I knew exactly what had happened," says Deb. "Eli laid back in my arms drooling. He could not sit up. He was dazed and not himself."[4] Deb told the teacher to call the hospital and tell them they were on their way. At eight years of age, Eli, born with sickle cell disease, had experienced an event usually associated with elderly people. He had had a stroke.

Sickle cell disease, sometimes called sickle cell anemia, is an inherited disease in which a mutation, or genetic mistake, exists in the gene that tells the body how to make a kind of protein called hemoglobin. Hemoglobin is the chemical substance in every red blood cell that allows the red cells to carry oxygen from the lungs to all the other cells of the body. It also allows the red cells to carry carbon dioxide back to the lungs so that it can be exhaled. Normal adult hemoglobin is called hemoglobin A, or Hb A. When the sickle cell mutation is inherited, the child's body makes a defective form of hemoglobin, called hemoglobin S, or Hb S. The "S" stands for "sickle." Hb S can cause red blood cells to change their shape and texture from soft and round to hard, sticky, and crescent-shaped. These sickle cells can cause episodes of severe pain, organ damage, stroke, and many other symptoms and complications. Treatment for the symptoms is

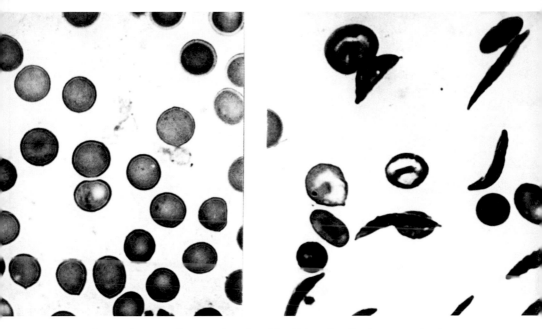

These photos of normal and sickled blood cells show marked differences.

available, but, as with many inherited diseases, in most cases there is no cure.

Genes and Sickle Cell Disease

One mutation in one gene is all it takes to cause sickle cell disease. Genes are extremely small chemical particles that exist in the nucleus of almost all living cells, plant or animal. They are made of a chemical called deoxyribonucleic acid, or DNA. DNA is like a code or a blueprint. The structure of an organism's DNA determines the structure and function of all the cells in the organism. There is a gene for every individual physical and behavioral characteristic of an organism. Genes are arranged along threadlike structures called chromosomes. Each cell nucleus contains forty-six chromosomes, twenty-three from each parent, so two genes for each characteristic are passed on.

Most genes are either dominant or recessive. If a gene is dominant, a child need only inherit one gene for that trait in order for the child to show that trait. If a gene is recessive,

Combinations of Dominant and Recessive Genes

B = brown eyes (dominant)
b = blue eyes (recessive)

Mother

	B	b
B	BB (brown)	Bb (brown)
b	bB (brown)	bb (blue)

Father

Odds of having a brown-eyed child: 75%

For a trait to be inherited, only one dominant gene is needed from either of the parents or two recessive genes, one from each parent.

the child must inherit it from both the father and the mother in order to show the trait. Eye color is a simple example. The gene for brown eyes is dominant, while the gene for blue eyes is recessive. If a child has blue eyes, it means he must have inherited a blue-eye gene from both of his parents. A brown-eyed child, however, may have one gene for brown eyes and one for blue eyes. He has brown eyes because the brown-eye gene is dominant.

The gene involved in sickle cell disease is called the hemoglobin beta, or HBB, gene, and it is located at one end of Chromosome 11. Its job is to provide instructions for making a certain part of the hemoglobin molecule. If the HBB gene contains a mutation, a disorder of hemoglobin will result. Sickle cell disease is just one of several disorders that result from mutations in the HBB gene.

The mutant HBB gene is a recessive gene, so people who have the disease have inherited a defective gene from each parent. They are said to have SS disease. People who inherit the sickle gene from only one parent (one Hb A gene and one Hb S gene) are said to have sickle cell trait rather than sickle cell disease. The genes that are inherited will determine how the child's red blood cells will behave for the rest of his or her life.

Sickle Cell Trait

If a child inherits only one gene for sickle cell disease, the child carries the trait for sickle cell disease but usually does not have symptoms of the disease. Sickle cell trait is found in about 8 to

People with sickle cell may have many different combinations of traits.

Sickle Cell Gene Combinations

Hb A = normal hemoglobin (dominant)
Hb S = abnormal, sickle-cell hemoglobin (recessive)

	Mother	
	HB A	**Hb S**
HB A	normal blood	sickle cell trait
Hb S	sickle cell trait	sickle cell disease

Father

10 percent of African Americans and, like sickle cell disease, is also seen in people of Middle Eastern, Caribbean, Indian, Italian, and Hispanic descent. About 3.5 million Americans carry the sickle cell trait.

People with sickle cell trait have hemoglobin type AS. Their bodies make both normal Hb A and abnormal Hb S. They may have some sickle cells in their blood, but they do not usually have symptoms of sickle cell disease and can lead normal lives. When they do have symptoms, the symptoms are milder than in people with the disease, and usually occur only under conditions of low oxygen, such as being at high altitudes, or under extreme physical stress, such as being very cold, very dehydrated, or out of breath from overexertion. On rare occasions, these low-oxygen conditions can trigger more severe symptoms or even sudden death.

Some people with sickle cell trait may have trouble concentrating their urine. This means that their kidneys excrete too much water. A small number may have some bleeding in their urine—a sign called hematuria. This is usually not serious, but a few individuals with hematuria may lose enough blood over time that they need medical attention.

People with sickle cell trait can pass their Hb S gene on to their children. If two people with the trait have a child, there is a 25 percent chance that their child will inherit the gene from both of them and have sickle cell disease. There is also a 25 percent chance that the child will inherit two normal genes and not have either the disease or the trait. There is a 50 percent chance that the child will inherit one normal gene and one defective gene, and that child will have sickle cell trait like his parents.

Sickle Cell Disease

Children who inherit both genes for sickle cell disease will show the symptoms of the disease. There are several different forms of sickle cell disease that can be passed from parent to child. Hemoglobin SS disease is the most severe form, in which the child inherits Hb S from both parents. In Hemoglobin

SC disease, the child inherits one sickle cell gene (S) and one gene for hemoglobin C (Hb C), another form of defective hemoglobin. SC disease is similar to SS disease, but the symptoms are much milder because Hb C does not cause sickling of the red cells as readily as Hb S. A third form of the disease is called sickle-beta thalassemia, in which the child inherits one sickle cell gene and one gene for another related blood disorder called beta thalassemia. The symptoms of this form of the disease can be mild or more severe and similar to SS disease. All forms of sickle cell disease, however, directly affect the red blood cells and the hemoglobin inside them.

Red Blood Cells and Hemoglobin

Hemoglobin is the protein inside red blood cells that allows them to carry oxygen. It is responsible for giving blood its red color. There are normally three types of hemoglobin in each

Three different types of hemoglobin are in each red blood cell: Hb A, Hb A2, and Hb F.

Types of Hemoglobin and Genes that Affect Hemoglobin Production			
Type	**Name**	**What It Is**	**What It Does**
Hb A, Hb A2	Hemoglobin A	Normal adult hemoglobin	Allows red blood cells to carry oxygen throughout the body from the lungs
Hb F	Fetal hemoglobin	Hemoglobin made by babies before and just after birth	Holds oxygen very tightly and is largely unaffected by SS disease; is replaced by Hb A and Hb A2 about 6 months after birth
PFH	Persistent Fetal Hemoglobin	Genetic mutation that occurs in some people with SCD	Allows certain individuals to retain and keep producing Hb F into adulthood
Hb S	Hemoglobin S	Defective hemoglobin that causes sickling	Makes red blood cells hard, sticky, and crescent-shaped
Hb B	Hemoglobin Beta gene	Gene located on Chromosome 11	Gene that, when mutated, can result in hemoglobin disorders
Hb C	Hemoglobin C	Defective hemoglobin	Milder form of hemoglobin disorder; does not cause red cells to sickle as readily as Hb S

red cell: Hb A, Hb A2, and Hb F, or fetal hemoglobin. Fetal hemoglobin is the kind that babies make before and just after they are born. It holds onto oxygen very tightly because babies in the womb do not breathe but get all their oxygen from their mother. In newborns, Hb F accounts for about 50 to 80 percent of the baby's total hemoglobin. As the baby grows, the Hb F is gradually replaced by Hb A or Hb A2. By six months, Hb F makes up only about 8 percent of the total. After six months, almost all the Hb F is replaced by adult hemoglobin.

Red blood cells, also called erythrocytes, are made in the bone marrow, the spongy, brownish-red material inside many of the larger bones of the arms, legs, spine, and hips. Their lives begin as stem cells, cells that have not yet become specialized into any particular type. Stem cells have the ability to become any kind of cell. The bone marrow releases stem cells according to need; if the body needs more red cells, stem cells are released from the marrow, converted to red cells, and sent into the bloodstream.

Normal red cells are smooth and round. They look somewhat like a donut without the hole in the middle. They are soft and flexible, so they can pass easily through even the tiniest blood vessels. Unlike some other types of cells in the body, red cells cannot reproduce themselves. Once they leave the bone marrow, they live for only three to four months. During that time, they circulate throughout the body, carrying life-giving oxygen to all the other cells in the body. At the end of their life span, they break apart in a process called hemolysis, and the hemoglobin inside them is recycled and used to make new red cells.

There are about 250 million red cells in a single drop of blood, and each cell contains about 265 million molecules of hemoglobin. Ninety percent of the total weight of a red cell is from the hemoglobin inside it, and carrying hemoglobin is its main job. Normal hemoglobin stays dissolved in the liquid part of the red cell. Iron atoms in the dissolved hemoglobin bind chemically with oxygen molecules (O_2). A molecule of hemoglobin can carry up to four oxygen molecules at a time. The red cells bring oxygen, brought in by the lungs during inhalation,

One Tiny Change

In the late 1940s, Nobel Prize–winning chemist Linus Pauling became interested in sickle cell disease. He knew that red cells sickle when oxygen levels are low, so he thought the problem might have to do with hemoglobin. He developed a way to tell whether a person had the disease or the trait by using a process for separating chemicals called electrophoresis. This technique could separate normal from abnormal hemoglobin, so Dr. Pauling was able to show that there were different kinds. In 1956, in the same laboratory where the structure of DNA had been discovered, another scientist named Vernon Ingram built upon Dr. Pauling's work with the goal of discovering exactly what the key difference was between the normal and abnormal forms of hemoglobin.

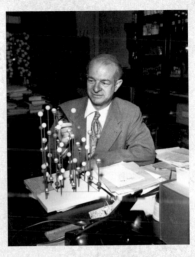

Dr. Linus Pauling developed a technique to separate normal from abnormal hemoglobin.

Like other proteins, hemoglobin is made up of chemical building blocks called amino acids. Hemoglobin's amino acids are arranged in four long chains—two alpha chains and two beta chains. Dr. Ingram used special chemicals to break up the hemoglobin chains into shorter pieces. Using electrophoresis, he compared the sequence of amino acids in both normal and abnormal forms of hemoglobin. He discovered that the only difference between the two was a change in a single amino acid. The amino acid valine was in the spot along the chain where glutamic acid should have been. This one tiny mistake is all it takes to change Hb A into Hb S and cause the devastating symptoms of sickle cell disease.

to all the other tissue cells to be used in carrying out their particular functions. They exchange the oxygen for two molecules of carbon dioxide (CO_2), a waste product of metabolism. The carbon dioxide is then carried in the red cells back to the lungs, where it is exhaled, and fresh oxygen is picked up.

Sickle Cells Are Different

When the sickle cell mutation exists, the baby's fetal hemoglobin is replaced by the abnormal Hb S rather than by Hb A. The defective Hb S can pick up oxygen in the lungs as well as Hb A, but it cannot hold onto its oxygen as tightly. When Hb S loses its oxygen, the abnormal hemoglobin molecules become undissolved, stick together, and turn into rigid, rod-like crystals condensed polymers. The longer the red cell is without oxygen, the longer the polymers grow. Polymerized hemoglobin causes the red cells to change their shape and texture. They become long, pointed, and crescent shaped, like a sickle used for cutting wheat. They also get hard and sticky. These abnormal red cells cannot carry oxygen like they should, so the body's cells do not get the oxygen they need. To make matters worse, the sticky, crescent-shaped cells can get stuck in smaller blood vessels, further cutting off blood flow and oxygen supply to the body's tissues. One geneticist explains:

> A red blood cell containing Hb A is like a filled water balloon at room temperature. It can easily be squeezed and bent. A red blood cell containing Hb S, on the other hand, is like a water balloon that has spent a few hours in the freezer. It is not flexible, it cannot be bent, and there is no way it can be squeezed through a tube that is narrower than the balloon itself.[5]

A number of factors can cause Hb S to polymerize, which in turn causes the red cells to sickle. The most important of these is the concentration of oxygen in the blood. In situations of low oxygen, the Hb S molecule loses its oxygen and polymerizes.

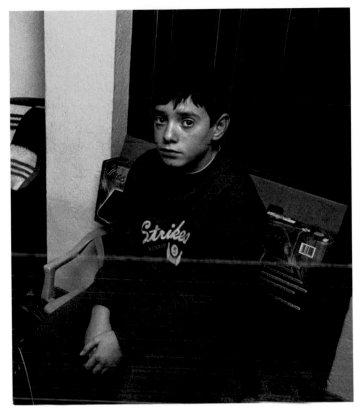

Fatigue, paleness, and shortness of breath are common symptoms of anemia.

Smoking is a major cause of low oxygen levels in the blood. It damages the lung tissue and prevents oxygen from being absorbed into the bloodstream. Being at high altitudes, such as mountain climbing or flying in unpressurized aircraft, can also cause low oxygen levels and trigger sickling. Lung diseases such as asthma, pneumonia, or respiratory infections can interfere with oxygen absorption. Temperature extremes, especially getting too cold, can trigger sickling because cold causes blood vessels to constrict, making it more difficult for sickled cells to move through them. Being cold also stimulates the body to increase metabolism in order to maintain body temperature. Increased metabolism uses up more oxygen.

Overexertion and getting out of breath during exercise can also cause sickling to occur, not only by causing low oxygen levels, but also by causing a condition called acidosis. Acidosis is a chemical imbalance in the blood in which the blood becomes more acidic than is normal. Acidity is measured by a number called the pH. Normal blood pH is about 7.4. A pH below that is considered acidosis. Acidosis can also be caused by inadequate intake of fluids, stress, smoking, alcohol consumption, diseases of the kidney, or diabetes.

If the sickled red cell gets exposed to oxygen again, the polymerized Hb S can become dissolved once more and the red cell can resume its normal shape. After many sickling episodes, however, or after long ones, the red cell's delicate membrane can be so damaged that it cannot regain its shape. The damage is irreversible, and the deformed cell is destroyed. Sickle cells die much sooner than normal red cells—after only ten to twenty days. This makes it difficult for the bone marrow to replace them quickly enough. The result is a significant shortage of red cells in the blood that leads to a condition called anemia.

Anemia

Anemia, which literally means "without blood," is basically a condition of inadequate hemoglobin. When there are too few red cells in the blood, or when the cells that are present cannot carry oxygen properly, anemia results. Sickle cell disease is often called sickle cell anemia because this symptom characterizes the disease more than any other, and all sickle cell patients experience at least some of the effects of anemia.

There are many different causes for anemia. A diet poor in iron can interfere with hemoglobin's ability to carry oxygen. Lack of proper vitamins, proteins, and fats can affect the bone marrow's ability to manufacture red cells. The marrow can also be affected by infections, drugs such as those used in chemotherapy for cancer, or other chemical factors such as lead poisoning. Red cells can be lost because of bleeding caused

Sickle Cell Trait and Malaria

The ethnic groups and nationalities in which sickle cell disease appears most commonly tend to come from tropical or sub-tropical areas of the world. The reason for this was unclear until the 1940s, when Dr. E.A. Beet, a British doctor in Rhodesia (now called Zimbabwe), in southern Africa, noticed that children with sickle cell trait did not suffer as much or die as often from malaria, a very common and often fatal mosquito-borne disease seen mostly in warm, moist, tropical areas. Dr. Beet found that the blood of malaria patients who also had sickle cell trait did not contain as many malaria parasites as other malaria patients. The sickle cell trait seemed to provide some sort of protection from malaria. Dr. Beet wrote about his observations, and soon other doctors began to see the same pattern.

For reasons that are not fully understood, the malaria parasite does not seem to survive as well in people with sickle cell trait. It may be that sickle cells do not carry enough oxygen for the parasites to survive. Another reason may be that sickle cells are destroyed by the spleen too rapidly for the parasites to repro-duce. A third reason has to do with the way sickle cell disease changes the chemistry inside the red cell, making it difficult for the parasites to survive.

Because people from tropical areas who have the sickle cell trait survive malaria more often, they live longer—long enough to have children and pass on the sickle cell trait. This helps explain why the two diseases share very similar geographic distributions and why sickle cell appears more often in these groups.

by illness, surgery, or severe injury. In sickle cell disease, the anemia is caused by an inadequate amount of normal, healthy red cells circulating in the bloodstream.

Fatigue, or extreme tiredness and weakness, is the main symptom of anemia and one of the most common symptoms of sickle cell disease. People who are anemic feel tired and worn out much of the time because their bodies' cells are not getting enough oxygen. In its most advanced stages, anemia can make it impossible for people to work, play, go to school, or concentrate. Terence, a young man with sickle cell, was unable to finish college because of fatigue. "I got tired just trying to walk around campus," he says. "I would get halfway to class and have to stop and take a half-hour break just to catch my breath."[6]

People who are very anemic may look pale. Their fingernails and the insides of their eyelids and cheeks may look lighter than usual. The sclera, the white part of the eye, may have a bluish tinge to it. If anemia goes untreated, later signs may include headache, dizziness, or fainting due to lack of oxygen to the brain, rapid heartbeat as the heart tries to pump more blood to the body, and shortness of breath as the lungs try to bring in more oxygen.

Anemia is a major symptom of sickle cell disease, but it is only one of many. Besides the symptoms that begin early in life and continue through childhood, sickle cell disease can lead to several long-term complications that affect many other body systems.

CHAPTER TWO

Symptoms and Complications

One of the mysteries of sickle cell disease is why symptoms vary so much among individuals. Even members of the same family who have the same disease may experience it in very different ways. Sickle cell disease affects most of the body's systems, so there are many different kinds of symptoms associated with it. Some symptoms are little more than minor annoyances. Some are more severe and may require hospitalization. Other symptoms and complications can be life-threatening emergencies. Some people go through life relatively healthy, while others need frequent hospitalizations. Though the reasons for this are not entirely clear, there are several genetic factors that are known to have an influence on the disease.

Genetic Influences

One of the genetic factors that influences the symptoms of sickle cell is the particular type of hemoglobin that is inherited and the amount of each type present in the blood. People who inherit two Hb S genes (SS disease) tend to have the most severe form of the disease and therefore tend to have more severe and more frequent symptoms. Another abnormal form of hemoglobin, Hb C, may be inherited along with an Hb S gene (SC disease). Hb C does not polymerize as readily as does Hb S, so the more Hb C that is present in a person's blood, the milder their symptoms are. These people may not even realize they have the disease for several years. People with the third type of sickle cell disease, sickle-beta thalassemia, have one Hb S gene and one gene for beta thalassemia, a disorder that affects the amount of hemoglobin produced. Their symptoms vary depending on how much normal hemoglobin they make.

Another genetic influence on sickle cell symptoms involves fetal hemoglobin, Hb F, which is the form of hemoglobin made in the unborn baby. Hb F holds onto oxygen very tightly and does not polymerize even if the baby has inherited SS disease. After birth, however, Hb F is gradually replaced by whatever form of adult hemoglobin has been coded for in the genes, whether normal or abnormal. Symptoms of sickle cell disease usually start to appear after about four to six months of age because this is the age at which much of the protective Hb F has been replaced by the abnormal Hb S. Some people, however, have a genetic mutation that allows them to continue making Hb F long after they are born and even into adulthood. This is called Persistent Fetal Hemoglobin, or PFH.

Hb S does not polymerize as easily when Hb F is present, even if most of the hemoglobin is Hb S. As one researcher describes it:

> It's like children's building blocks with pegs and holes in them—you could make a big tall tower of them. That's just what happens with sickled hemoglobin. A whole string of them get stuck together. But fetal hemoglobin doesn't have the peg or the hole.[7]

The PFH mutation, therefore, provides some protection for the person who has it, and symptoms are milder. Sheila, an adult with sickle-beta thalassemia, has the PFH mutation.

> We, my husband and I, learned that my high level of fetal hemoglobin had and has continued to serve as an antidote to frequent and severe crises. Yes, I have experienced many crises throughout my life; however, I believe that I have been spared perhaps more crises and associated

health decline due to having this Super Baby Blood as I call it. Due to the PFH, I have been blessed to lead a very productive life.[8]

Sheila is lucky to have the PFH mutation. It has provided her with at least some protection from one of the most serious and painful of sickle cell symptoms, the sickle cell crisis.

The Sickle Cell Crisis

The sickle cell crisis, or sickling episode, is one of the most dramatic of sickle cell symptoms in both children and adults. A sickling crisis occurs when Hb S in the red cells loses its oxygen, polymerizes into crystals, and becomes hard and rod-like. This forces the red cell to change its shape from soft and round to stiff and crescent shaped. When the sickled cells get stuck in a blood vessel and cut off the oxygen supply to an organ or joint, this is called an infarction and results in a painful crisis.

A person suffering an acute sickle cell crisis may need to be hospitalized.

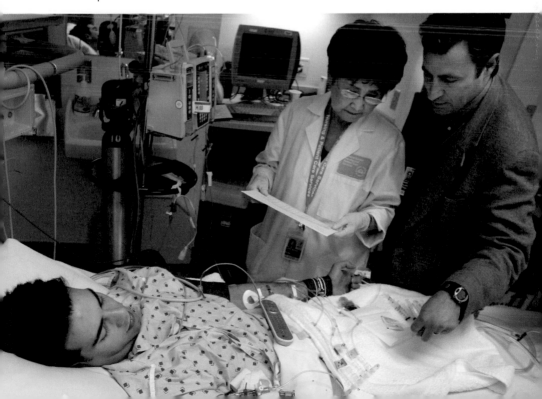

Differences Between Thalassemia and Sickle Cell

Thalassemia is not a single disease but is actually a group of diseases that, like sickle cell disease, are caused by recessive mutations that affect hemoglobin. It is seen most commonly in people of Middle Eastern, Asian, and Mediterranean descent. The major difference between thalassemias and sickle cell disease is that the mutations that cause thalassemia produce a deficiency of hemoglobin rather than a mutant form of it. Thalassemia does not cause sickling.

Hemoglobin is made up of four molecule chains: two alpha chains and two beta chains. Four genes are needed to make alpha chains, and two are needed to make beta chains. Thalassemias are classified according to which chain is affected, alpha or beta, and how many of their genes are mutant or missing. There are four kinds of alpha thalassemias and three types of beta thalassemias. Sickle-beta thalassemia, a form of sickle cell disease, results from a combination of beta thalassemia and hemoglobin S—the kind of hemoglobin found in sickle cell disease.

Symptoms of thalassemia can range from mild to severe, depending on the particular type of thalassemia inherited and how much of each hemoglobin chain is made. One form causes no hemoglobin at all to be made; infants born with this form cannot survive after birth. Symptoms are very similar to those of sickle cell disease: anemia and fatigue, enlargement of the spleen, and bone problems. Crises do not occur because the red cells do not sickle as in sickle cell disease. As with sickle cell, treatment depends on the symptoms and involves frequent blood transfusions.

If the oxygen supply is not restored quickly, the affected tissue can become inflamed, causing more pain and possibly a fever.

Repeated infarctions can cause permanent damage to the organ tissue. Pain episodes are most often felt in the chest, abdomen, lower back, shoulders, knees, hips, and thighs.

Like other symptoms of sickle cell, the experience of the crisis can be very different from person to person. Some sickle cell patients may not have a crisis for several years at a time, some may have only one or two crises in a year, and others may have as many as fifteen or more. Acute, or short-term, episodes usually last for a few hours; longer ones may last for days or even weeks. Between episodes, patients are usually pain-free, though they may feel very tired and may have some numbness or tingling in the affected area. Some individuals may experi-

A person with sickle cell disease may become jaundiced if the bilirubin builds up.

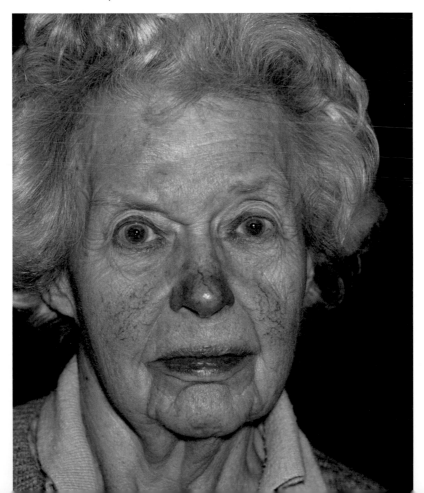

ence chronic, or long-term, pain that can last several months or even years. Still others may have a combination of both acute and chronic pain. Some crises can be managed at home with pain medications such as acetaminophen or codeine; others may require a trip to the hospital to get them under control with more powerful medications such as morphine, given directly into the bloodstream. Sickle cell crises can happen very suddenly, and it can be difficult to predict when and where one will occur.

Acute Chest Syndrome

Acute chest syndrome is a sickling crisis that occurs in the lungs. It is similar to pneumonia. Symptoms may include fever, chest pain, coughing, and difficulty breathing. Several factors contribute to acute chest syndrome. The chests of sickle cell patients tend to be smaller than normal. At the same time, their hearts tend to be enlarged because they have to work harder than healthy hearts to get oxygen to the rest of the body. This means that there is less room for the lungs to expand, and less air is inhaled with each breath. When a sickle cell patient gets an infection in his lungs, the decreased oxygen level may trigger an episode. Blood vessels in the lungs can get blocked by sickled cells and also trigger an episode. Severe acute chest syndrome is the most common cause of death in sickle cell patients, so a person with these signs should be taken to the hospital right away. Repeated lung infections and episodes of acute chest syndrome can lead to permanent lung damage in older sickle cell patients.

Abdominal Crises

As with acute chest syndrome, sickling episodes and infarction involving the organs in the abdomen can cause severe pain and organ damage. Two organs in the abdomen that are particularly vulnerable are the liver and the spleen.

The liver is a large, dark reddish-purple organ located in the upper right side of the abdomen, just below the rib cage. It has several functions related to metabolism, excretion of waste products, and digestion. When sickled red blood cells become trapped in the liver, the person feels pain in that part of the abdomen. The person may also become jaundiced. Jaundice is a yellowish discoloration of the skin and the whites of the eyes caused by the buildup in the blood of a waste product called bilirubin. Bilirubin is produced when red blood cells are destroyed. It is normally excreted from the body by the liver. Because sickle cells break apart and die so fast, often there is too much bilirubin present in the blood, and the liver cannot excrete it fast enough.

Splenic Sequestration

Like the liver, the spleen is very vulnerable to the effects of sickling. The spleen is located in the upper left side of the abdomen, near the stomach. It is also dark red but is smaller than the liver. The spleen filters out damaged and abnormal red blood cells. It also has a very important role in the immune system. In the spleen, cells called phagocytes destroy bacteria and remove other unwanted particles from the blood. The spleen also produces antibodies—chemicals that attack foreign material such as viruses. A person with an unhealthy spleen has more trouble fighting off infections than someone with a healthy spleen.

Sickled cells often get stuck in the spleen because it is a highly vascular organ, meaning it has a great many small blood vessels in it that divide into many tiny branches. When sickled cells get trapped in the spleen, it swells and causes pain. Sometimes the spleen becomes chronically enlarged, and more and more blood can get trapped inside it. Enlargement of the spleen can show up as early as two years of age. Long-term swelling damages the spleen so that it cannot work as well.

When a large percentage of the body's red cells get trapped in the spleen in a short period of time, the spleen swells very quickly, causing a severe pain episode called splenic sequestration. Besides intense abdominal pain, patients experiencing this type of crisis may also have profound anemia, rapid heartbeat, dizziness, fever, or difficulty breathing. When this happens, the

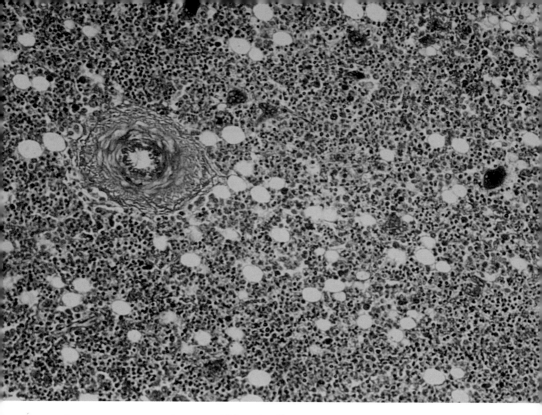

Bone marrow produces red blood cells.

patient must be hospitalized and have a blood transfusion. The mother of a two-year-old girl with sickle cell disease describes her child's experience:

> She went to bed one night and her tummy was hurting her. And the next morning … her stomach was really big, like when you see people in Africa who haven't been eating. It was really big and real hard. So I rushed her to the hospital.… And she was in a lot of pain, a lot of pain! She would run high-grade fevers of 103, she wouldn't eat or drink, she had hardness in the stomach and pains in her legs.… They found out she had an enlarged spleen.… That's what makes her stomach real, real hard.… And if you touch it, or she moves, she just screams.[9]

Sometimes, the only way to prevent this from happening again is to remove the spleen, a surgical procedure called a splenectomy. People can live without the spleen, but splenec-tomy is a last resort because the patient then loses all the immune functions of the spleen and becomes even more prone to infections. More infections often mean more crises.

After years of damage and tissue death in the spleen due to inadequate blood supply caused by sickled cells, the spleen may actually begin to shrink in size. As early as the teen years, the shrinking spleen may disappear altogether. This phenomenon is known as auto-splenectomy, meaning that the body literally "removes" the spleen itself. As with surgical splenectomy, the individual loses all the immune system benefits of the spleen and may become more prone to infections

Sickle Cell Crises in the Bones and Joints

The bones are another common site for the symptoms of a sickle cell crisis. Besides providing the human body with support and protection, the bones are responsible for producing the stem cells that are converted into red blood cells as they are needed. Because sickle cells die off and are destroyed so quickly, the bone marrow of a sickle cell patient is especially active and must have an adequate oxygen supply of its own in order to function.

When a sickling episode occurs in the bones, the bone tissue does not get its oxygen. When this happens, the patient experiences swelling and pain in the bones and joints and may get a high fever. As a result of the infarction, the bone marrow may stop producing new red cells, a serious event called an aplastic crisis. If the marrow does not eventually resume red cell production, the patient will die. Ingrid, a woman in her mid-forties with sickle cell disease, describes her experience: "The aplastic crisis racked my body with so much pain that I can only describe it as feeling like I had been hit with a runa-way freight train. This aplastic episode was also accompanied by high fevers in excess of 105 degrees."[10]

The location of bone pain can change as a person grows. In very young children, it often occurs in the hands and feet. In older children, it tends to be in the arms and legs. In teens and adults, pain may occur in the shoulders and hips. Back pain is common as well. When pain occurs in the bones, it tends to happen on both sides of the body at once.

Hand-Foot Syndrome

The sickle cell pain that occurs in the hands and feet of the very young child is called hand-foot syndrome. Often, this is the first symptom that a child has, appearing anywhere from six months to two years of age. It is rarely seen later in life. Tiny blood vessels in a baby's hands and feet can easily become blocked by sickled cells. They may swell and become very painful. The swelling often begins on the backs of the hands and feet and then moves into the fingers and toes. Rapid and painful swelling can also occur in the bone marrow cavities of the small bones of the hands and feet and cause damage to the bones. Hand-foot syndrome may also involve a fever. It is treated by giving the child pain medication and fluids.

Infections and Fevers

Besides hand-foot syndrome, young sickle cell patients are also more prone to getting infections because of the damaging effect the disease has on the spleen. This damage also makes it harder to get rid of an infection once it has started. Infections caused by bacteria are the most common cause of death in children under five who have sickle cell disease. One bacterium in particular, called *Streptococcus pneumoniae* (commonly known as strep), causes many infections in younger children. The most serious strep infections occur in the blood (septicemia), in the membrane surrounding the brain (meningitis), and in the lungs (pneumonia). Strep infections in the bones and joints can be very painful and difficult to treat. Bladder and kidney infections are also common.

Fever is often an early symptom of an infection because it is a sign that the immune system is trying to fight off the infection. Low-grade fevers of less than 100 degrees are often not treated because they can have a beneficial effect in fighting infections. Sometimes, however, the body temperature can rise much higher, as high as 105 degrees or more. This is a danger- ous situation because high fevers can cause seizures in chil- dren. For this reason, it is important to take the child to the doctor whenever a fever develops so that the cause of the fever can be pinpointed and treated.

As the young sickle cell patient grows into the school-age years, hand-foot syndrome and splenic sequestration become less frequent problems. After about age ten, fevers and infec- tions also occur less often. As the child grows older, however, other symptoms and complications become more frequent. One of the most severe is a potentially life-threatening compli- cation called stroke.

Stroke

The brain is like the command center for the entire nervous system. It controls thought processes, learning, movement and coordination, memory and personality, and the functioning of all the other systems in the body. Although it makes up only 2 percent of the total weight of the human body, it accounts for about 20 percent of the body's total oxygen consumption. The brain must get the oxygen it needs if it is to remain healthy and function normally. A stroke occurs when a part of the brain, for any reason, does not get enough oxygen. Severe brain damage or even death can be the result.

Sickle cells do not carry as much oxygen as normal red cells, so the body compensates for this by sending more blood to the brain in an effort to get more oxygen to it. The added pressure of this extra volume of blood in the brain can cause severe headaches in the sickle cell patient. If the pressure of the extra blood becomes too great, blood vessels in the brain can rupture, or break, causing bleeding inside the brain. This kind of stroke is called an intracerebral (inside the brain) hem- orrhage and is seen more often in older children and adults. When this happens, the broken blood vessel cannot deliver its blood supply to the brain tissue that it feeds, so that area of the brain is deprived of oxygen. Blood is very irritating to the brain tissue and disrupts the normal chemical balance in the brain.

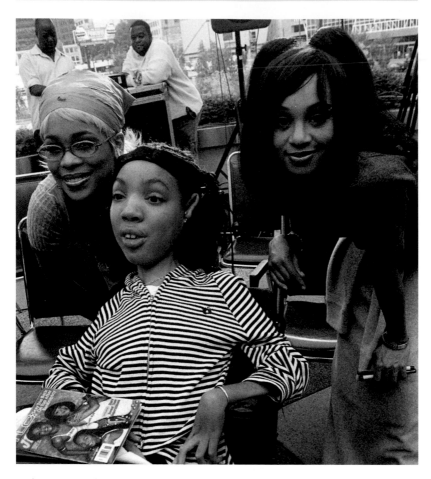

Ischemic strokes occur in about 11 percent of sickle cell patients by the time they turn twenty years old.

In addition, the build-up of free blood in the brain can exert pressure on the surrounding tissue, and damage to that part of the brain can occur if the pressure is not relieved quickly.

In younger sickle cell patients, a different type of stroke, called an ischemic stroke, is more common. Ischemia is a condition that results when tissue cells do not get the oxygen they need and begin to die. An ischemic stroke happens when an artery in the brain becomes blocked and blood cannot get to the part of the brain fed by that artery. In sickle cell disease, sickled cells can easily block off an artery and cause ischemia,

"A Brain Attack"

Hippocrates, an ancient Greek who is known as the Father of Medicine, first recognized stroke over 2,400 years ago. At that time, it was called apoplexy, which is Greek for "struck down by violence." It was so named because the symptoms came on very suddenly, and people affected would become paralyzed or have changes in their behavior.

Centuries later, in the mid-1600s, Dr. Jacob Wepfer discovered, through dissection of corpses, that people who had died from apoplexy had had either bleeding or a

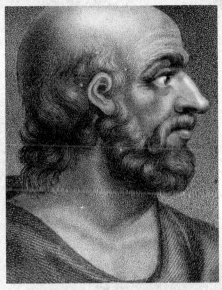

Hippocrates, the Father of Medicine, first recognized stroke more than 2,400 years ago.

blocked blood vessel in their brains. In 1928, apoplexy was divided into categories based on the cause, and the terms "stroke" and "cerebral vascular accident" (CVA) were used to refer to it. Today, stroke is often called a "brain attack" because it is caused by an interruption of blood flow to the brain, much as a heart attack is caused by interrupted flow to the heart.

A great deal is known today about the causes, treatment, and prevention of stroke. Most stroke victims have a good chance for survival and recovery if they are treated right away.

or lack of blood supply, to the brain. Ischemic strokes occur in about 11 percent of sickle cell patients by the time they turn twenty years old.

Symptoms of a stroke can come on very suddenly, or they may develop gradually. The person may complain of a bad headache. He or she may have visual disturbances, weakness or loss of feeling on one side, or difficulty speaking. A severe stroke may cause convulsions and unconsciousness. Depending on the kind of stroke suffered, the amount of brain tissue damaged, and the way the stroke is managed after it happens, recovery may be fast or very slow. Recovery is sometimes complete, with no permanent effects. Other strokes may cause permanent visual or speech problems, paralysis of one side of the body, coma, or death.

Other Complications

Sickle cell crises, splenic sequestration, aplastic crises, and strokes are all emergencies that require immediate medical attention. There are other symptoms, however, that, although not life-threatening, can be major problems for sickle cell patients. These complications involve several different body systems.

Gallstones

One body system affected by sickle cell disease is the biliary system, which includes the gallbladder and the bile ducts that lead from it into the small intestine. One of the by-products of red cell destruction is a chemical called bilirubin. Bilirubin is excreted by the liver in a sticky, brownish-green liquid called bile. Bile is stored in the gallbladder, a small, pouch-like organ located just underneath the liver. The gallbladder stores bile until a meal is consumed. Then it squeezes the bile out into the small intestine, where it helps with digestion of fatty foods.

In sickle cell disease, unhealthy red cells are destroyed at a very rapid rate, and a great deal of bilirubin is produced. The liver cannot keep up, and the excess bilirubin in the bile can contribute to the formation of small stones in the gallbladder. A very common problem in adults, gallstones can form even in young children who have sickle cell disease. Gallstones can block the ducts that lead out of the gallbladder so that the gall-bladder cannot squeeze the bile out. This can cause abdominal pain and nausea, especially after eating fried or fatty foods. The symptoms of gallbladder disease tend to get worse as time goes by, and surgical removal of the gallbladder is often necessary.

Skin Ulcers

The skin can also be damaged by the effects of sickled cells. When blood supply to the skin is disrupted because of blockage in the small capillaries, the skin can break down and develop sores called ulcers, especially on the lower legs and ankles. Common in older adults, especially those with diabetes, skin ulcers in sickle cell patients can appear as early as the teen years. They may develop after an injury that breaks the skin, or they may just appear spontaneously. Skin ulcers are painful and can get infected easily. They are hard to treat because a healthy blood supply is necessary for proper healing of any tissue. Even

Skin ulcers are a common and painful effect of sickle cell disease.

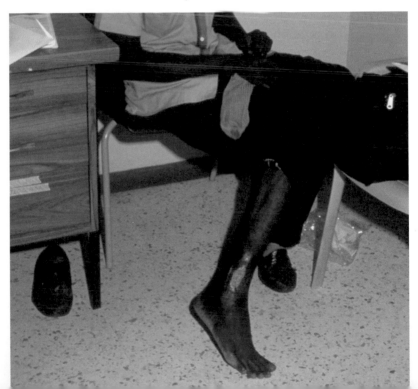

after they heal, which can take months or even years, the scar tissue left behind can break down again and cause new ulcers.

Late Complications

Some effects of sickle cell disease show up later in the patient's life. In adulthood, acute pain episodes are not as common as they were in the childhood and teen years, but chronic, almost constant pain can be a major problem. Repeated sickling episodes in the bones can lead to sickle cell–related arthritis and necrosis, or breakdown, of the hip or shoulder joints. One sickle cell researcher who herself has sickle cell disease says:

> I had my most severe painful episodes when I was younger, but it has evolved into a chronic type of pain that I have just about all the time. It's similar to arthritis, but instead of just my joints hurting, the whole bone itself hurts.... When I feel it coming on, I try to engross myself in my work and ward it off. I don't always succeed.[11]

Strokes, the threat of which diminishes in the teen and young adult years, become more of a threat once again later in life. Also, repeated sickling episodes over the years can cause damage to several other organ systems because of oxygen deprivation and scarring of the organ tissue. The kidneys and lungs are particularly susceptible to long-term damage.

CHAPTER THREE

Diagnosis and Treatment

Because sickle cell disease is a genetic disorder, a diagnosis can be made before a child is even born. At birth, before symptoms begin, newborns who are at risk for having the sickle cell gene can be screened, or tested, to see if they carry one or two sickle cell genes. Once the diagnosis is established, measures are taken to help prevent, minimize, or treat symptoms. Treatment and prevention measures begin very early and continue throughout life.

Prenatal Counseling

Couples who have any form of sickle cell disease, or who know the trait is in their families and wish to have children, may want to have genetic testing done to determine whether or not they carry the trait and what the chances will be that their children will inherit the disease. If both husband and wife are found to have the trait, they can seek prenatal counseling from a genetic specialist to learn more about the disease and what life is like for a sickle cell child and the family. Some counseling centers introduce couples to patients with sickle cell who can tell them firsthand what their lives are like. Couples can then make a more informed decision about starting their families.

Newborn Screening

In the late 1960s, many African Americans felt that the U.S. government was ignoring the needs of sickle cell patients for racial reasons. In response, President Richard Nixon approved massive funding for sickle cell research. The disease gained national attention, and plans for newborn screening programs were made.

The first newborn screening programs for sickle cell disease were begun in the 1970s. Massachusetts was the first state to start regularly screening newborns who were at risk for having sickle cell disease. Unfortunately, many of these programs were incomplete and poorly planned, and they did not include adequate education for the public. Also, many people questioned why screening was even necessary. There was no cure for the disease, and screening could not prevent it. Because only African Americans were screened, many people of other groups who had the disease were missed. One study conducted in North Carolina found that newborn screening programs targeted only toward African Americans were missing about 20 percent of children with sickle cell disease. By the end of the decade, many of these screening programs had ended.

In 1987, the National Institutes of Health recommended that all newborns, regardless of ethnicity, be screened for sickle cell disease so that a minimum of cases would be missed. Research has since shown that early detection and treatment is critical for the well-being and survival of children with sickle cell disease. As of 2006, forty-seven states had mandatory universal screening programs for sickle cell disease.

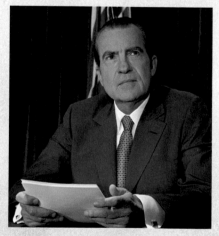

President Richard Nixon approved funding for sickle cell research.

Prenatal Testing

Couples who are at risk for having a child with sickle cell and decide to have a baby may choose to have the baby tested before it is born. This serves two purposes. First, it provides freedom from worry for the parents if their baby is found to have inherited normal genes. Second, if the baby does have the disease, it gives the parents and other family members time to learn more about it and how to manage the child's health after it is born. It also allows time for them to prepare emotionally and financially for the extra needs of a sickle cell child.

Prenatal testing of a baby's genes is most often done in one of two ways. Chorionic villus sampling, or CVS, is a test that can be done as early as ten weeks into the pregnancy. In this test, a tiny tube is inserted through the mother's vagina and into the womb. There is no discomfort to either the mother or the baby. Tissue cells from a part of the placenta called the chorionic villi, which have the same genetic make-up as the baby, are removed through the tube. The genes in the cells are examined to determine whether or not the baby has inherited the suspected disease.

The other method for obtaining tissue for genetic testing is amniocentesis. This procedure is usually done at about fifteen to eighteen weeks. In this procedure, an anesthetic is injected into the skin of the mother's abdomen. A long, very thin needle is inserted through the abdomen and into the womb. A small amount of amniotic fluid, which surrounds and cushions the baby, is withdrawn. In the amniotic fluid are cells that have been shed by the baby. The cells are then examined for genetic defects.

Newborn Screening

Both CVS and amniocentesis are highly accurate in determining whether or not a child has inherited sickle cell disease or sickle cell trait. After the child is born, the diagnosis is confirmed by direct examination of the baby's blood, taken either from the umbilical cord immediately after birth or from a heel stick. This may also be done if there is a family history of sickle cell disease but prenatal testing has not been done. Newborn screening is

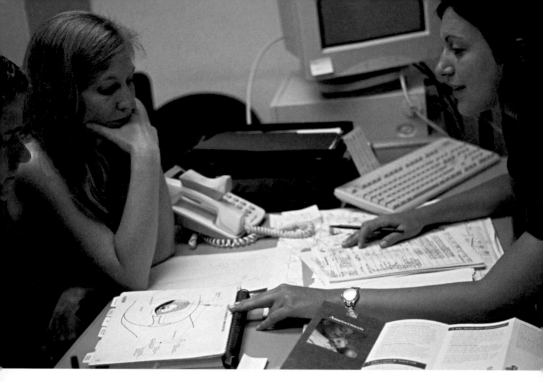

Couples who have sickle cell disease in their families may want to have genetic testing before having children.

very important in confirming a diagnosis early in life so that preventive measures can be started as soon as possible, before the protective fetal hemoglobin is replaced by adult hemoglobin. Today, most states have universal screening programs so that every baby born is automatically tested for sickle cell.

Several blood tests are available that can confirm the diagnosis. Children who have a positive result are retested to ensure the accuracy of the results.

Hemoglobin Electrophoresis

Hemoglobin electrophoresis is the most commonly used diagnostic test. This test separates out and measures the different types of hemoglobin present in a person's red blood cells. The term "electrophoresis" refers to the movement of an electrically charged particle through a gel when it is subjected to an electric field. The electric field is created by placing a positively charged electrode at one end of the gel and a negatively charged electrode at the other end. When large protein molecules such as hemoglobin are placed in the gel and subjected to the electric field, they will migrate, or move, through the gel toward either the positive electrode or the negative electrode, depending on their own electrical charge. Different kinds of hemoglobin carry different electric charges, and each type moves in different ways through the gel, separating them from one another. The molecules are then stained so they can be seen. They appear as bands of different widths spread out from one end of the gel to the other. In this way, the different types of hemoglobin in a person's blood can be identified and the amount of each can be measured.

Isoelectric Focusing

Isoelectric focusing is very similar to electrophoresis in that the hemoglobin molecules are placed in gel and subjected to an electric current, but this method relies on the fact that a molecule's electrical charge will change depending on the pH, or acidity level, of the surrounding gel. In isoelectric focusing, the gel is more acidic at one end than at the other. As the hemoglobin molecules move through the gel under the influence

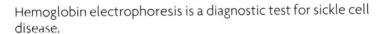

Hemoglobin electrophoresis is a diagnostic test for sickle cell disease.

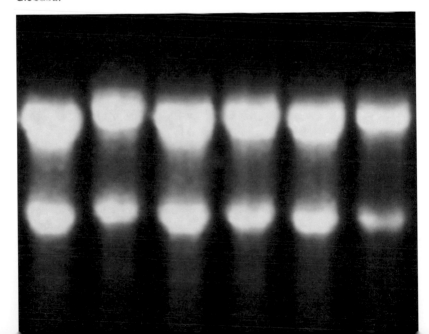

of the electrical field, their electrical charge changes with the changing acidity of the gel. When a molecule reaches the part of the gel where the gel's pH causes the molecule to lose its electrical charge, it stops moving. In this way, the hemoglobin types are separated, or focused, into sharp bands, and the amounts of each can be measured.

High-Performance Liquid Chromatography

This test, simply referred to as HPLC, also separates different types of hemoglobin from one another, permitting measurement and analysis. In HPLC, the hemoglobin is dissolved in a gas or liquid solution. The solution is then forced through a tube that has been tightly packed with material that absorbs the solution. Different molecules dissolve in the material differently. The more absorbable the molecule is in the material, the longer it will take to travel through the tube. The less absorbable it is, the quicker it will travel through the tube. HPLC is very precise and can separate proteins like Hb S and Hb A that only differ by a single amino acid.

Other Blood Tests

When the diagnosis of sickle cell disease has been confirmed, the patient is referred to a hematologist, a doctor who specializes in disorders of the blood. The hematologist will order further tests to evaluate the severity of the disease, monitor its progression, check for possible complications, and evaluate the effects of treatment. These tests are repeated regularly throughout the life of the patient.

The complete blood count, or CBC, is a simple and frequently done blood test that can be used to check for anemia, the presence of infection, and many other conditions. It measures the amounts and characteristics of the various kinds of cells and other components of the blood. It provides information about the different types of white blood cells (part of the immune system), the number and size of the red cells and the amount of hemoglobin in them, and the number of platelets (necessary for blood clotting). It also measures the hematocrit, which indicates the percentage of space the red cells take up in the blood. Sickle cell patients typically have a low red cell count, low hemoglobin, and low hematocrit. They may have a high white cell count, which often indicates an infection somewhere in the body.

Other tests are done that may show abnormal results in the sickle cell patient. If a patient has jaundice, a yellowish

Other blood tests are used to check for anemia, infection, and other conditions.

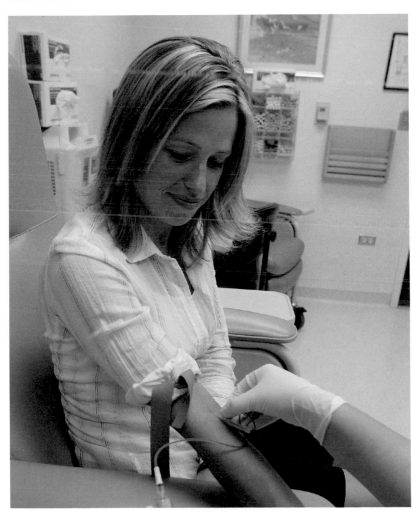

discoloration of the eyes and skin, the amount of bilirubin in the blood may be elevated. This is an indicator of possible liver damage or gallbladder disease. Elevated serum creatinine and potassium, as well as blood cells in the urine, indicate possible kidney damage.

Treatment

After the diagnosis and blood tests, prevention measures begin immediately. "The most important visit is the first visit," says a doctor from Georgia.

> You have a fine line between scaring people to death about this beautiful new baby they have and making them respectful—but not afraid—of this disease. I tell parents their babies couldn't have been born at a better time and place because of everything that is available to them to intervene. There have been so many research advances.[12]

The goals of sickle cell treatment focus on preventing crises, relieving symptoms when they occur, and preventing or minimizing complications. Treatment and prevention methods encompass a wide range of strategies, including diet and hydration, medications, blood transfusions, and oxygen therapy. For some fortunate individuals, stem cell transplants are an option that offers hope for cure.

Diet and Hydration

Proper diet and good hydration are simple but extremely important measures that a sickle cell patient can take to prevent and minimize symptoms. A healthy, well-balanced diet is important for all children, but it is even more so for children with sickle cell disease. Research has shown that sickle cell children need as much as 20 percent more calories than other children. The extra calories are needed to provide the energy necessary to make new red cells, help prevent infections, carry out daily activities, and grow at a normal rate.

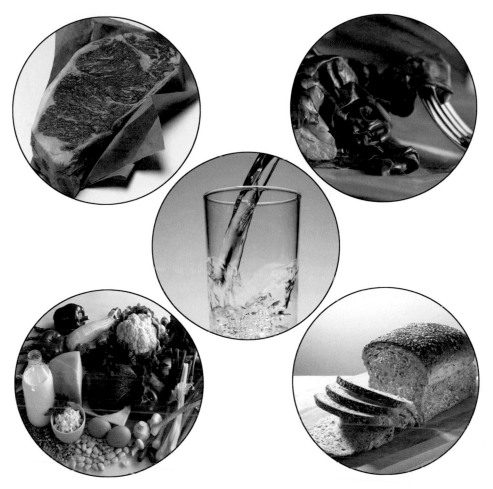

Good diet and hydration are absolutely essential for people with sickle cell disease.

Several nutrients are especially important for sickle cell patients. Folic acid is a type of vitamin B found in leafy vegetables, grains, and fruit. It helps the body to produce red cells more quickly. Iron is the mineral in hemoglobin that binds to oxygen so that the red cells can carry it. Iron is found in dark leafy vegetables like spinach and in whole grains, beans, dried fruit, and red meats. Vitamin C helps the body to absorb iron more efficiently. It also helps prevent and fight infections. The doctor will decide if the child should take extra supplements of these nutrients.

One of the simplest but most important things a sickle cell patient can do to ward off painful crises is to drink lots of fluids. Drinking even a small amount of extra water every day can significantly decrease the number and severity of crises. There are several reasons for this. First, when a person becomes dehydrated, the volume of liquid in the blood is decreased. This means that the cells in the blood become more crowded. Sickle cells are already sticky and tend to clog up blood vessels, causing a crisis. When they are crowded closer together in a dehydrated person, a crisis becomes even more likely to occur. Staying well hydrated keeps the cells from sticking to one another and helps the blood flow more smoothly. Second, adequate hydration keeps the red cells themselves full of fluid. When Hb S molecules come into contact with one another, they polymerize, causing sickling. Adequate fluid in the red cell keeps the Hb S from becoming too concentrated in the cell. A third reason to stay well hydrated is to help offset the higher-than-normal loss of water that results when damaged kidneys cannot concentrate the urine properly. People with sickle cell disease can become dehydrated very quickly because of this. Last, drinking extra water can help to alleviate a pain episode that is already happening, and it also helps to control the body temperature during a fever.

Medications

In addition to proper diet and hydration, medicines are a part of everyday treatment for many sickle cell patients. Medications for sickle cell disease help to treat and prevent infections, manage pain, prevent sickling, and improve blood flow.

To prevent and treat infections caused by bacteria, doctors prescribe antibiotics. Infants born with sickle cell disease start taking the antibiotic penicillin as soon as the diagnosis is made. The goal is to prevent potentially deadly infections like pneumonia, which causes many sickle cell deaths in infancy and early childhood. Children take penicillin every day until about age five, when lung infections are not as great a threat. If the child is allergic to penicillin, as many people are, another antibiotic called erythromycin may be used. Antibiotics also help adult patients avoid infections and treat them if they occur.

A vaccine is a medication that not only prevents people from contracting a disease but actually makes them immune to the disease, meaning that they cannot get it. Starting in infancy, children in the United States routinely get vaccines for several diseases, such as measles, mumps, rubella, tetanus, and others. Children with sickle cell disease may be given another vaccine called pneumococcal conjugate vaccine, or PCV. This vaccine prevents infection by the microbe pneumococcus, which can cause meningitis, flu, or the liver disease hepatitis. Pneumococcal disease is one of the leading causes of death in sickle cell children.

Children with sickle cell disease are given a number of vaccines to prevent infections.

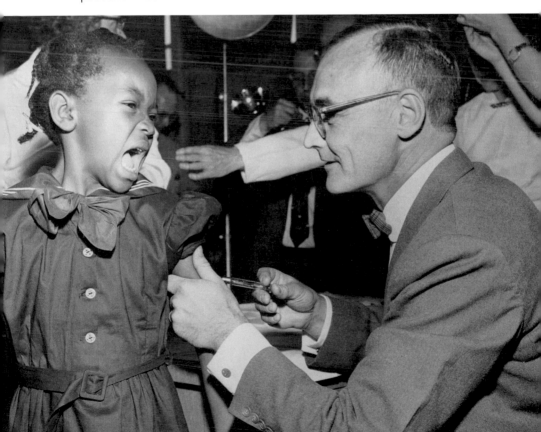

The vaccine seems to be changing that, however. A study published in June 2007 reported that, since 2000, when PCV was introduced, the rate of serious pneumococcus diseases dropped by more than 90 percent in children under age five. "I was not surprised that there was a decrease," says the director of the study, "just surprised about the magnitude of the decrease."[13]

Pain Medications

Like antibiotics and vaccines, pain medications are a frequent part of life for sickle cell patients. Depending on their severity and location, milder pain episodes may be managed by over-the-counter medications such as acetaminophen or ibuprofen. More severe pain may require a prescription medication such as codeine or hydrocodone. For the most painful crises, hospitalization may be necessary so the patient can be given strong narcotic painkillers such as morphine, given as injections or directly into the bloodstream through an IV.

Hydroxyurea

One drug that has been shown to be particularly effective for preventing painful crises is hydroxyurea. Hydroxyurea was originally developed as a cancer treatment. In the mid-1990s, researchers found that it could dramatically increase the amount of protective fetal hemoglobin in adult sickle cell patients. The frequency of sickle cell crises, particularly acute chest syndrome, was decreased by about 50 percent for patients in the study, and the need for hospitalizations and blood transfusions was also cut in half. A follow-up study showed that the drug also helps sickle cell patients live longer compared with patients who do not take the drug.

The way it works is not yet entirely clear, but it seems to work by suppressing bone marrow activity. When the more active bone marrow stem cells are suppressed, the less active marrow cells, the ones that produce stem cells with Hb F genes, become more active. One sickle cell expert explains, "We think that hydroxyurea works, at least in part, by turning back on the production of fetal hemoglobin in adult sickle cell patients."[14]

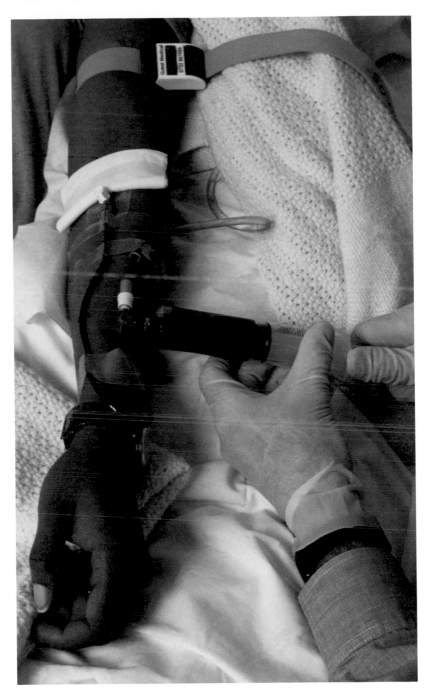

Blood transfusions are given to treat severe anemia.

It also seems to help prevent red cells from sticking to the sides of blood vessels and clogging them up.

Blood Transfusions

In addition to medications, blood transfusions are a frequently used treatment method for sickle cell patients. A blood transfusion involves giving a person blood that has been donated by another person. The blood is given over several hours through an IV directly into the patient's bloodstream. Blood transfusions are given to treat severe anemia by increasing the number of healthy red cells in the circulation.

In children with sickle cell disease, blood transfusions are given to counteract the sudden, severe anemia that can occur during splenic sequestration or acute chest syndrome. Regular monthly transfusions can also help prevent strokes, especially in children who have already had at least one stroke. Transfusing blood helps by diluting the concentration of sickle hemoglobin with cells that contain normal hemoglobin.

Lloyd, a British teen with sickle cell disease who had a stroke when he was eleven, goes into the hospital once a month to get a blood transfusion to minimize his chances of having another stroke. Lloyd has made a video about his experience getting the transfusions. He says:

> One day a month I go into Great Ormond Street Hospital's sickle cell unit and have a blood transfusion. I have one to two pints of blood which can take three to four hours. It can get boring while I'm having the blood transfusion. I'll try and watch some TV, play computer games or watch a video. The main thing I don't like is the time it takes to have the transfusion. I could be doing something else instead. But I know it's something I have to have so it's hard to say I don't like being in hospital because I know the transfusion helps me.[15]

Although blood transfusions are very helpful when given for the right reasons and can be life-saving, there are several

U.S. Blood Type Percentages

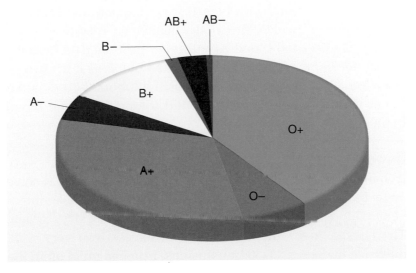

The blood types of both the donor and the patient must match closely.

possible complications associated with them. One of these is transfusion reaction. A blood transfusion is similar to an organ transplant in that living tissue (the red cells) from one person is given to another person. The donor's blood type must be compatible with, or closely matched to, the blood type of the patient. If the donor blood is not compatible, a transfusion reaction occurs, which is similar to a severe allergic reaction. Health care providers who transfuse blood watch the patient very closely for signs of a transfusion reaction. Signs can include mild itching and pain at the IV site, blood in the urine, and respiratory arrest.

Fluid overload can happen if the transfusion is given too quickly and the body does not have enough time to adjust to the added volume in the blood vessels. Too much volume administered too quickly can actually cause an intracerebral hemorrhage, and it can stress the heart as it tries to pump the extra volume. If the larger volume of blood cannot get through the vessels, it may flow too slowly and possibly cause a pain episode.

Alloimmunization is a problem that can happen after repeated transfusions in which the body begins to recognize even compatible donated blood as a foreign protein. The immune system kicks in and attacks the donated blood as if it were an infection. The immune system creates antibodies to donated blood, making it more difficult to find compatible donor blood in the future.

Blood Transfusions and Iron Overload

Iron overload is a major concern for patients who must receive many blood transfusions. The mineral iron is a normal component of blood and is necessary for hemoglobin to carry oxygen. The human body does not get rid of excess iron very well, however, and after 20–30 transfusions, iron can build up in the body and cause poor growth; damage to the heart, the endocrine glands, and the liver; and even sudden death. One physician explains, "If you give one unit [about 300cc] of blood, you are giving 250 milligrams of iron. Considering the fact that in many cases you do this repeatedly, you are adding a significant amount of iron."[16] The patient's total body iron level is monitored closely to prevent this, but if it happens, the extra iron must be removed.

Iron Chelation

The process for removing excess iron is called iron chelation. A medicine called a chelating agent is given by injection into the tissue under the skin over a period of eight to ten hours overnight for five nights. Iron binds chemically to the chelating agent and is then excreted in the urine. The urine can take on a pink color as the iron is excreted. The downside of this therapy is that it is not well tolerated by most young patients, and it can be difficult to persuade children and their parents to stick with it.

Exchange Transfusion

One way to avoid iron overload is with a procedure called exchange transfusion. Exchange transfusion is a therapy in which donor blood is transfused while, at the same time, sickle blood is removed. Healthy blood is exchanged for sickle cell blood. This can be done during emergency situations when the concentration of sickle cells must be decreased quickly. It also helps prevent fluid and iron overload.

Stem Cell Transplant

Austin Jones was diagnosed with sickle cell disease shortly after birth. From infancy, he suffered many complications from his disease, including bone infections, pneumonia, acute chest syndrome, and at least one stroke. He needed blood transfusions every three weeks. "All of this told us that Austin had a severe form of sickle cell disease, meaning that he was vulnerable to limb- and life-threatening strokes, infections, and lung and heart damage later life," says his doctor.[17] The doctor discussed with Austin's parents the possibility of a bone marrow transplant.

Bone marrow is the soft, spongy material inside the larger bones that is responsible for producing stem cells, which the body can convert into red blood cells as needed. The bone marrow stem cells in sickle cell patients become red cells that carry Hb S, but if the bone marrow is replaced with healthy marrow, the person can start making cells with normal Hb A. A stem cell transplant is currently the only way that sickle cell disease can be cured.

As with blood transfusions, the marrow donor's tissue must be a very close genetic match to the patient's, or else the patient's immune system will reject the donor marrow. The best donor is a brother or sister, especially an identical twin, whose tissue exactly matches the patient's.

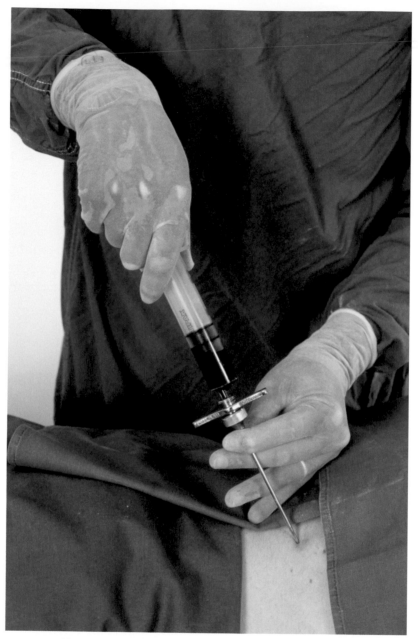

A stem cell transplant is currently the only cure for sickle cell disease.

The procedure for bone marrow transplant begins by giving patients very powerful drugs that effectively destroy their own marrow cells and inhibit their immune systems so that their bodies will not attack the donor marrow. This is called myelo-ablation. When myeloablation is complete, the donor is pre-pared for the donation.

In the past, marrow donation required minor surgery under anesthesia to draw the marrow out of the hip bone. Today, the most common method does not actually involve removing any marrow at all, but it is still commonly called bone marrow donation. In this procedure, stem cells are filtered directly out of the donor's blood. The donor is given once-a day injections of a drug that stimulates the release of stem cells from his mar-row into his bloodstream. After several days of injections, the donor goes in for the donation. A special machine draws blood from the donor's arm and separates out the stem cells in a pro-cess called apheresis. The rest of the blood is returned to the donor. The donated stem cells are then infused into the reci-pient. Within ten to twenty days after the infusion, the donor cells move into the bone cavities, take the place of the patient's destroyed marrow, and become red cells that contain normal hemoglobin.

Bone marrow transplant carries with it some significant risks. The drugs given to the patient before the transplant are very toxic and can cause side effects such as diarrhea, mouth sores, or damage to the lungs or liver. Until the patient's immune system resumes function, which can take as long as two months, the patient is at high risk for infections. A major concern is graft-versus-host disease (GVHD), in which the donated marrow actually attacks the patient's organs as if they were foreign protein. If this happens, more drugs must be given to further suppress the immune system. If the patient's system rejects the donor marrow, the transplant may fail. Other major issues include finding a compatible donor and the cost of the procedure, which is considerable.

The National Marrow Donor Program

The earliest experiments in bone marrow transplantation were done in France in the late 1950s, when researchers discovered that it seemed to work in mice. A breakthrough came in 1958 when a French researcher discovered proteins called human leukocyte antigens, or HLAs, found on the surface of most of the body's cells. HLAs can distinguish between cells and proteins that belong to a person and those that do not. When HLAs recognize a foreign substance, the immune system forms antibodies to try to destroy it.

After the HLA system was discovered, researchers worked to learn how it could be used to match donors with recipients and help prevent rejection, or graft-versus-host disease. Until then, only identical twins could safely donate marrow to each other. By the 1960s, physicians had learned enough about the HLA system to try transplants between non-identical siblings. The first successful transplant of this kind was done in 1968 at the University of Minnesota. By the 1970s, doctors had learned enough that transplants between unrelated people became possible. The first unrelated marrow transplant was done in 1973 at Memorial Sloan-Kettering Hospital in New York City.

In the late 1970s, health professionals began to develop the idea of a national bone marrow registry, a database that would provide a list of volunteer donors who had been HLA-typed. In this way, potential donors all over the country could be quickly identified for patients who did not have a suitable match in their family. In 1984, Congress passed the National Organ Transplant Act, which provided funds to establish such a registry. The National Bone Marrow Donor Registry began operations in July 1986. In 1988, the name was changed to the National Marrow Donor Program.

Austin was lucky. His older brother was a good match, and at the age of five, he received his transplant. "We're very excited at the idea that Austin's battles with pain, infections, pneumonia, and blood transplants are behind us," says his father. "It seems like we've spent the majority of his life in doctor's offices or hospitals. This bone marrow transplant will give Austin a chance to be a normal five-year-old, and to grow to be an old man."[18]

CHAPTER FOUR

Living with Sickle Cell Disease

In 2004, a study done at the University of Texas Southwestern Medical Center proved what medical professionals had long suspected—that sickle cell patients were living longer, getting fewer fatal infections, and dying less often from the disease than ever before. "Research developments during the past several decades have improved the lives of many persons with sickle cell disease," says the study's senior author. "It was only a half century ago that very few persons with sickle cell anemia and related conditions survived beyond twenty-one years of age."[19]

Living with sickle cell disease has improved dramatically in the last three decades because of the great strides that have been made in the understanding of the disease and its treatments. Although stem cell transplant is, as yet, the only hope for cure, the pain and disability brought about by the disease are today much more manageable. Early diagnosis, prompt and thorough medical care, and meticulous home care make the difference.

Sickle cell disease has a profound impact not only on the life of the patient but also on the lives of the parents, siblings, friends, teachers, and everyone else involved in the child's life. Frequent pain, fatigue, the need for many medications, frequent doctor visits and hospitalizations, and restrictions on activities are a part of everyday life. Preventing symptoms and

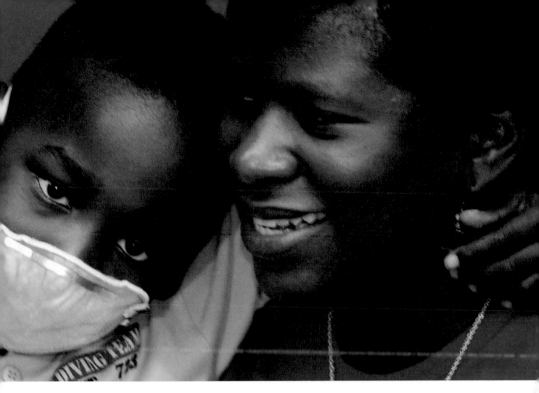

Sickle cell disease has a great impact on everyone in the child's life.

complications requires daily adherence to a strict plan of care. Emotional and psychological support for the patient and family are as important as medical support. Proper management of this very complex disease requires the coordinated efforts of many health professionals.

Physicians

A variety of specialists may be involved in the sickle cell patient's care throughout the course of his life. One of the first to see the patient is the hematologist, a doctor who specializes in disorders of the blood. Some hematologists specialize further in the treatment of sickle cell disease. They work mostly in sickle cell treatment centers located in larger cities. Pediatricians also get involved very early in the child's life. These physicians specialize in the care of children and often coordinate the care provided by other specialists. Family practice physicians work with both children and adults and may also coordinate care. Internists are doctors who work with the medical problems of adults. They assume the care of the patient upon reaching adulthood. Obstetricians and gynecologists specialize in the needs of women and will help care for the adult female sickle cell patient during pregnancy. Nephrologists and urologists manage any urinary tract problems, including kidney disease, which may arise because of sickle cell. When necessary, surgeons and anesthesiologists will be involved in providing anesthesia and surgery to remove a diseased gallbladder or spleen or to repair a damaged joint. Emergency physicians work in hospital emergency rooms and evaluate and care for sickle cell patients when they have to come to the ER.

Other Caregivers

Besides physicians, many other caregivers are involved in the care of the sickle cell patient. Nurses care for patients when they are in the hospital and may also visit the patients at home. Nurses provide a wide range of services twenty-four hours a day, including education, counseling, dressing changes, and medications. They keep a close eye on the patient, keeping track of fluid intake and nutrition, monitoring vital signs, watching for signs of pain episodes and complications, and communicating closely with the doctors.

Physical therapists work with the patient to help maintain or improve muscle strength and flexibility after surgery, injury, or a bone crisis. They teach patients ways to help manage pain and keep their joints as healthy as possible.

Chronic, debilitating diseases such as sickle cell can have a profound emotional and psychological effect on both patients and their families. Children in particular can become very stressed, anxious, and depressed because of the constant fear of pain and illness and the restrictions on the things they can do. Stress itself is a known trigger for sickle cell crises, and the pain leads to even more stress. Children and teens with sickle cell often feel left out and isolated from their peers because of their disease. Psychiatrists and psychologists provide counseling to help people cope with the stresses of being chronically ill. Psychiatrists can prescribe medication, if necessary. Psychologists are not physicians, but they can teach patients how to use different methods such as biofeedback and relaxation techniques to help deal with pain. They can also help with any school and social problems that may arise.

Education

All of the health care professionals described can provide information for patients and families. This education is the very first line of defense in managing sickle cell disease. Sickle cell is a very complicated disease, and there is a great deal to learn. Education is necessary so that early signs of problems can be recognized and treated before they become unmanageable. Sickle cell organizations, treatment centers, and clinics can provide education as well as counseling to help patients and their families cope with the stresses of sickle cell disease.

Managing and Preventing Pain Episodes

One of the major goals of the sickle cell patient's medical team is to prevent and manage pain episodes. Pain is a frequent, almost daily occurrence for many people with sickle cell disease. Parents and children become very familiar with the signs of an impending crisis and learn to deal with them quickly. It can be difficult, however, for the parents of a very young child to know how much and what kind of pain the child is in if he is too young or in too much distress to communicate verbally. Deb Hill, the adoptive mother of eight-year-old Eli, has learned through experience how to know what her child is experiencing:

> A parent has to learn the facial expressions to determine the intensity of the pain. Ibuprofen can be given first; if it works you'll know by the expression. If ibuprofen doesn't work, then you try a high-powered prescription for pain. Again you look at the face. If the high-powered prescription pain reliever doesn't work, you get to the hospital immediately for morphine, fluid, and blood. It's the stages of facial expressions that you eventually learn that help you know what to do.[20]

The Oucher Scale

It may be difficult or impossible for very young children to communicate to a caregiver how much pain they are having during a sickling episode. It may be difficult for a caregiver to know whether or not the child needs to go to the hospital. In order to help young children communicate their degree of pain, the Oucher scale was developed in 1990 by Mary J. Denyes, PhD, RN, and Antonia M. Villaruel.

The Oucher scale shows a series of six children's faces. Each face shows a different expression of pain, starting with a calm face at the bottom of the scale and leading up to a screaming face at the top. Alongside the faces are the numbers 0 at the bottom through 100 at the top. Children or caregivers can match a face on the scale to what the child in pain is expressing and give the expression a number. For example, a child in some pain may look like a 20 or 30 on the scale, and a child in a great deal of pain may look like a 70 or 80. This helps the caregiver decide if the pain episode can be managed at home or school or if it is bad enough that the child may need professional medical attention for a more serious complication.

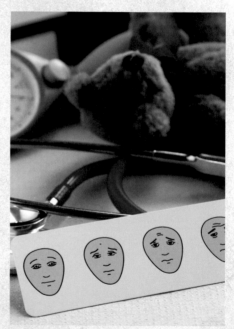

The Oucher scale was developed to help caregivers judge the degree of pain in very young children.

Fortunately, much is known about conditions that trigger these episodes. There are several things a sickle cell patient and his family can do daily to help prevent or minimize pain episodes.

Staying Hydrated

Keeping well hydrated is critical for preventing sickle cell crises. Water is the best fluid to drink, and it should be readily available throughout the day. It can be difficult, however, for a parent to get a child to drink a lot of water every day. Good alternative sources of fluid that even young children enjoy are fruit juices, caffeine-free soft drinks, popsicles, gelatin, milk, ice cream, soups, and watery fruits and vegetables like watermelon or tomatoes. People with sickle cell should avoid liquids that contain alcohol or caffeine. Both chemicals are diuretics; that is, they cause increased urine production and can cause the body to actually lose more fluid than is taken in, which leads to dehydration. In addition, when alcohol is metabolized in

It is critical for people with sickle cell disease to stay hydrated.

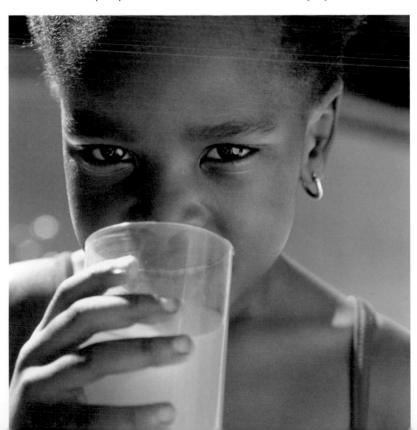

the body, it increases the acidity of the blood, which can trigger sickling. It also interferes with the body's ability to use B vitamins such as folic acid, and it is very toxic to the liver.

Activity and Rest

Just like healthy people, people with sickle cell disease need to exercise regularly in order to help prevent illness and maintain their strength and energy, but they must be very careful not to exercise to the point of exhaustion. Most doctors recommend that high-impact or high-contact sports be avoided. Activities such as walking and bike-riding can provide good exercise without overexertion. Children must be careful when they play

Regular, nonstrenuous exercise, such as bike riding, is important in maintaining strength and energy.

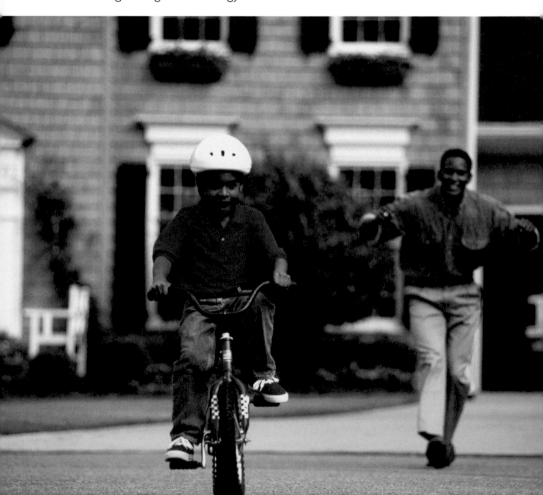

outside during very hot or very cold weather, as both temperature extremes can trigger a pain episode.

Adequate rest is also very important. The anemia of sickle
cell can cause a person to tire very easily. Overexertion can
overheat the body. It can also create a more acidic environment in the blood because working the muscles intensively
produces lactic acid. Being out of breath decreases the amount
of oxygen in the blood. All of these conditions can trigger a
crisis. For these reasons, children with sickle cell need to get
enough sleep at night and rest or take naps throughout the day
if they feel tired.

It is important for sickle cell patients to avoid situations and
places where oxygen is low. Activities such as scuba diving and
mountain hiking are examples of such situations. Traveling in
airplanes is safe as long as the aircraft is completely pressu-
rized to compensate for the altitude, but some types of smaller
aircraft may not be. If it is necessary to be at a high altitude for
any reason, the person may need to carry a portable oxygen
tank to help prevent a sickling crisis.

Avoiding Infections and Fever

Avoiding infections is another major issue in the daily lives of
sickle cell patients. Young children are particularly prone to
getting infections because of the damage the disease causes
to the spleen, which has a major role in the immune system.
Bacterial infection is one of the major causes of death in young
sickle cell patients. Early prophylaxis, or prevention, with daily
penicillin, getting a flu shot every year, and keeping up to date
with immunizations go a long way toward preventing infections. Meticulous attention to thorough hand washing helps
prevent the spread of bacteria and viruses between people.
Bathing regularly and maintaining a clean environment also
help to limit contact with infectious organisms. Regular dental
care keeps the teeth and gums healthy and helps prevent tooth
loss and infections in the mouth.

Fever is an early sign of an infectious process in the body. Whenever a sickle cell patient gets a fever, an immediate call to the doctor is in order.

Psychological Effects

The effects of sickle cell disease are more than just physical. Any chronic, lifelong illness also has psychological, emotional, and social effects. When that illness begins in very early childhood, as sickle cell disease does, these issues must be dealt with by the entire family.

The first people to have to deal with the emotional stresses of sickle cell are the parents of the affected child. Many parents, especially those who knew beforehand that they had the trait and could have a child with the disease, face feelings of guilt over having a child who will experience pain and discomfort for much of his or her life. Parents who are not aware that they had the trait may at first express disbelief that their child is ill. They may react with anger, depression, or hostility toward the doctors or each other. They may experience a great deal of anxiety over how they will handle the financial burdens of caring for their child.

It is very important that parents come to accept the reality of the situation, learn all they can about the disease, and focus on how to help their child. At the same time, however, it is important that they not become overprotective of their child. This can be harmful to the child because it may lead to feelings in the child of helplessness, weakness, and overdependence on others. A child's self-esteem can be reduced because of this. It is important for children with sickle cell to be treated as "normal" children as much as possible, with the same expectations of behavior at home and at school, so that they will not feel different and isolated from their siblings and friends. Della, a young man from Ghana who has sickle cell, says:

> When I was young, my family never knew when a teacher would turn up at their home with me in tow screaming, in a crisis. They were always worried about me, but I still

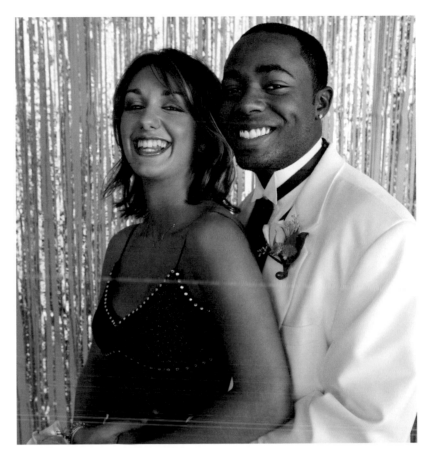

Children and teens with sickle cell disease should try to maintain much the same activities as their friends.

had to do my fair share of washing the dishes—I was never allowed to wallow in my condition or use it as an excuse.[21]

Besides parents, children and teens also have to deal with emotional aspects of chronic illness. The teen years are difficult for most people, but they may be especially difficult for teens with sickle cell. Independence from parents and acceptance by peers is very important to teens. They worry about getting jobs, dating, and future marriage. Having to deal with a chronic illness can interfere with all of these goals. Teens can get

"FARMS"

A simple way that even young children can remember the basic principles of prevention in sickle cell disease is to think of "FARMS":

F - Food, Fluids and Fever. Eat a well-balanced diet. Always remain well hydrated by drinking plenty of fluids, especially water, every day. At the first sign of fever, call the doctor.

A - Air. Try to avoid situations that may decrease the amount of oxygen in the blood, such as being at high altitudes, getting out of breath, and traveling in unpressurized airplanes. Have supplemental oxygen available if these situations are unavoidable.

R - Rest. Get enough sleep at night and take breaks and naps whenever you feel tired.

M - Medications and Medical Care. Take all prescribed medications as directed by the doctor. Follow closely the doctor's plan of care.

S - Situations. Be aware of certain situations that can cause problems, like getting too tired, too hot, or too cold. Avoid stressful situations as much as possible and know how to deal with them if they arise. Stay away from alcohol, caffeine, illegal drugs, and smoking.

depressed and frustrated. Parents and friends can help the teen with sickle cell to take a positive outlook. Despite having to get blood transfusions every month, Lloyd, a teen who lives in London, England, has a very optimistic attitude. "I won't let it stop me," he says. "I won't use it as an excuse. I just try to go on as normal as I can."[22]

Older brothers and sisters of a sickle cell child will have their own issues to deal with. They may come to feel that their younger sibling is taking from them the attention that they have been used to getting from their parents. They may show resentment or hostility toward the ill child because of this. The added financial burden on the family may mean that the healthy siblings must do without the kinds of toys, clothes, or other privileges they are used to. Balancing attention between an ill child and healthy siblings adds additional stress to the lives of the parents.

Most communities, especially larger cities, have support groups available for sickle cell patients and their families. These groups help parents and kids meet others who are dealing with the same issues and understand their feelings and experiences. Parent groups help their members with support, encouragement, and helpful tips for coping with specific situations. They also help each other with educational and financial resources. Peer groups for kids help their members develop positive ways of dealing with their disease and provide chances to meet other kids like them.

Family Planning

Because today's sickle cell patients are more likely than ever to live beyond childhood and into adulthood, planning their own families can be a major issue for them. For couples at risk of

A couple at risk may choose to adopt children.

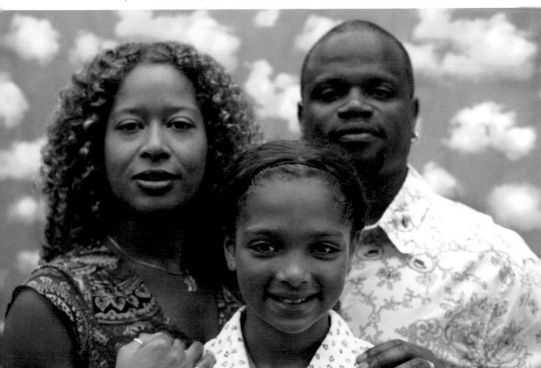

having a child with sickle cell disease, the choice of whether or not to start a family is a personal decision that requires good communication and a thorough understanding of the disease. Except for couples in which both have the disease, it is now possible for any at-risk couple to plan their family so that none of their children will be born with sickle cell disease, using methods of prenatal genetic testing and in vitro fertilization techniques. If they do not know whether or not they carry the trait, they may wish to have genetic testing to find out.

At-risk couples may want to meet with a genetic counselor before starting their families. The counselor can provide all the information necessary for the couple to make a fully informed decision about having children. Once they have learned about the disease itself, the financial and psychological issues involved, and what life is like for a child with sickle cell, they can decide whether or not they want to risk having a child with the disease. If they decide they do not want to take the chance, they have several options. They may decide not to have biological children of their own and perhaps adopt children instead. They may decide to start a pregnancy and have the fetus tested before birth using amniocentesis or CVS. If their child has SS disease, they must then decide whether or not to continue the pregnancy. This may be a very difficult decision for many couples to make due to religious or personal feelings about ending a pregnancy.

A third option is called in vitro fertilization with preimplantation genetic diagnosis, or PGD. This is an advanced technique that is very expensive and may not be an option for every couple. It involves removing egg cells from the mother and fertilizing them in a laboratory dish with sperm cells from the father. After the fertilized eggs begin to divide and grow into embryos, they are tested genetically for the sickle cell gene. Only the embryos that test negative for sickle cell disease are implanted into the mother's uterus where, hopefully, at least one will successfully develop into a healthy baby. In this way, at-risk couples can ensure that they will have healthy babies. The first successful use of PGD was in 1999, when two people who both had sickle cell trait gave birth to twins who were both free of the sickle cell gene.

Pregnancy and Sickle Cell Disease

When a woman with sickle cell disease becomes pregnant, there are special considerations for her health and the health of her baby. Women with sickle cell trait generally do not experience problems any more than a woman who does not have the disease at all. They may have more frequent urinary tract infections, however, and, like many other pregnant women, they may become anemic due to iron deficiency and need a dietary iron supplement.

Some women with sickle cell disease have no change in their disease during pregnancy. Others may experience more complications because of it. High blood pressure and severe anemia are the most common. Because of the extra volume of blood made during pregnancy, sickling episodes may occur

Careful monitoring is necessary for the pregnant woman with sickle cell, both for herself and the baby.

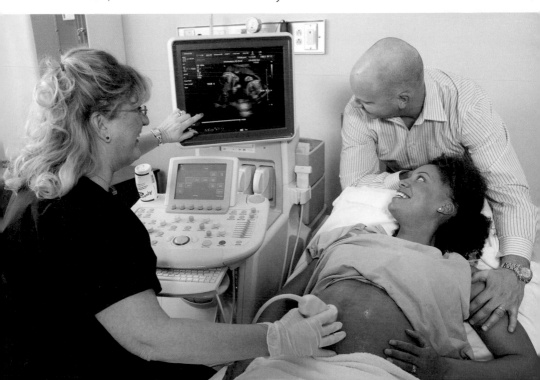

more often, and the heart may become enlarged from trying to pump the extra volume. Any organ damage that already exists may become worse during pregnancy. Gallbladder disease is fairly common during and after even normal pregnancies; it poses a particular risk to the mother with sickle cell.

There are added risks for the unborn child as well. During a sickling episode, the body may move blood away from the uterus in favor of more vital organs. This may deprive the fetus of oxygen and nutrients and cause it to grow more slowly than normal and to be smaller than normal at birth. Some expectant mothers may require blood transfusions during pregnancy to help ensure that the baby gets enough oxygen while in the womb. There is also an increased risk of miscarriage, premature delivery, and stillbirth.

Early and regular prenatal care is necessary for all new mothers but especially for the woman with sickle cell. Her doctor may want her to have more frequent visits so she can learn more about how to take care of herself and her baby and to closely monitor their health. Sickle cell mothers are almost always anemic at the time of the first visit. Iron supplements may be prescribed, but only after making sure that she is not iron-overloaded from previous blood transfusions. Besides the normal measures of a healthy diet and prenatal vitamins, it is especially important that she stay well hydrated to help prevent sickling. She may require IV fluids to prevent dehydration, especially if she struggles with morning sickness and loses fluid because of it. Her liver and kidney function will be watched closely during the pregnancy. During labor, she will most likely be given extra oxygen to breathe.

With thorough education and counseling, proper prenatal care, and careful monitoring, there is no reason a woman with sickle cell disease should not be able to have children. Except for some additional tests and precautions, care of the pregnant sickle cell patient is very similar to that of a healthy mother-to-be.

CHAPTER FIVE

On the Horizon

Today, there are many effective methods for the diagnosis and treatment of sickle cell disease, its symptoms, and its complications. Beyond today's methods, however, promising new trends are being researched. Current research focuses on using genetic knowledge to improve diagnosis and developing medications and other therapies that help alleviate pain episodes and prevent complications. The ultimate goal for the future is a cure for sickle cell disease that is safe, effective, and available to all patients.

Fine-Tuning Diagnosis

Methods for early diagnosis of sickle cell disease can distinguish the trait from the disease and can pinpoint which variation of sickle cell disease is present, but they cannot explain completely why the symptoms vary so much among individuals with the same disease. Using what is already known about human genetics, scientists are working to learn more about what genetic factors influence the way the mutation is expressed in individual people. They hope to someday be able to identify an individual patient's genetic "blueprint," one that can predict what specific symptoms and complications that particular person will tend to have. It may be possible to use that information to provide custom-made treatments that will prevent the complications before they even begin.

Medications

Ongoing research into new and existing methods of medical treatment has several goals. One is to reduce the concentration of defective hemoglobin in the blood by stimulating the body to make other kinds of hemoglobin, particularly fetal hemoglobin. Another goal is to get more oxygen to the affected areas during a pain episode by improving blood flow and helping sickled cells return to their normal shape. A third goal of treatment with medication is to make sickled cells less sticky and prevent them from sticking to blood vessel walls.

Research with Hydroxyurea

Research continues into more effective ways to use hydroxyurea, the anti-cancer drug that stimulates production of Hb F. The first studies on hydroxyurea were begun in 1991. The results of the initial research were so remarkable that the studies were stopped sooner than planned, and in 1998 the drug was approved by the Federal Drug Administration (FDA) to treat sickle cell disease in adults. Although it has not yet been officially approved for use in children, many treatment centers began using it almost immediately in teenagers and are now using it to treat young children and babies. In 1994, a study called the PED HUG confirmed that children between the ages of five and fifteen respond to hydroxyurea as well as adults, with increased levels of fetal hemoglobin, decreased pain episodes and hospitalizations, and decreased complications. The study also showed that hydroxyurea does not affect normal growth and development in these children. A later study, called the HUSOFT, looked at the effects of hydroxyurea in infants from six months to two years of age and followed their progress for several years. "The results of the HUSOFT trial showed that infants with sickle cell anemia not only tolerated hydroxyurea, but could benefit from it just as older children and adults do," says Winfred Wang, MD, director of the St. Jude Comprehensive Sickle Cell Center. "In addition, these infants may have had less organ damage and better growth than untreated patients."[23] A new study called the BABY HUG, now being conducted at several centers in the United States, will show if hydroxyurea can prevent long-term organ damage when it is started at a young age, between nine months and eighteen months. So far,

Sickle Cell Disease Medications			
Drug	How It Works	Benefits	Drawbacks
Hydroxyurea	Increases production of Hb F	Leads to decreased pain, fewer complications; does not affect normal growth	Suppresses production of white blood cells and platelets; can lead to certain types of cancer
Erythropoietin (and hydroxyurea)	Hormone that increases production of red blood cells in bone marrow	Use with hydroxyurea increases production of Hb F more than using either drug alone	Effect on patients with pre-existing kidney disease or pulmonary hypertension
Arginine butyrate (L-arginine)	Increases concentration of Hb F	Significantly increases fetal hemoglobin	Must be given intravenously, results not seen in all patients

Many medications are being studied for their impact on the treatment of sickle cell disease.

researchers are very optimistic. As one researcher says, "Oh my goodness, if a child is not doing well and we put him on hydroxyurea, it's like a new life. They eat well, they play well, they grow better, they have new energy, they see themselves as well. It's not the end-all answer, but, boy is it wonderful."[24]

Other research with hydroxyurea builds on earlier studies that looked at combining it with another drug called erythropoietin. Erythropoietin is a hormone, naturally made in the kidneys, that tells the bone marrow to increase production of red blood cells. Like hydroxyurea, it is commonly used to help cancer patients who are anemic because of chemotherapy. Giving erythropoietin along with hydroxyurea stimulates the production of fetal hemoglobin at a higher rate than using either drug alone does. The National Heart, Lung, and Blood Institute is studying how well this combination works in sickle cell patients who already have kidney disease or high blood pressure in the lungs, a dangerous condition called pulmonary hypertension.

Currently, hydroxyurea is the only drug approved in the United States for treating sickle cell disease. The drug does not work for everyone, however, and it has some negative side effects, such as suppressing normal bone marrow. It often causes nausea, especially in the first few weeks. Because it suppresses the bone marrow, it may also suppress the production of other desirable types of blood cells, such as white cells, a key part of the immune system, and platelets, which are necessary for proper blood clotting. It can also suppress red cell production too much, making anemia worse. With long-term use, it may cause leukemia or skin cancers to develop. It can cause genetic mutations, a concern for anyone wanting to have children. Also, it does not work in all patients. Doctors monitor dosages of hydroxyurea very closely, watching for these side effects and adjusting the dosage as necessary. Says one researcher, "Clearly, we need to develop safer and more effective drugs for sickle cell disease. By evaluating a variety of potential drugs, we hope to contribute to developing a range of drugs for different stages and different complications of the disease."[25] To that end, several other drug therapies that target specific aspects of the disease are being investigated.

Arginine Butyrate

Another drug that is being researched for its ability to increase the concentration of fetal hemoglobin is arginine butyrate, or L-arginine. Interest in this drug for treating sickle cell came after doctors noticed that babies born to diabetic mothers maintained production of fetal hemoglobin longer than babies born to non-diabetic mothers. Butyrate, a by-product of chronic high blood sugar, was found to be the explanation for this. Some early trials showed a significant increase in fetal hemoglobin, but this effect was not seen in all trials. A disadvantage is that it must be given intravenously. Research is underway to find ways to make arginine butyrate a more useful option.

One unexpected side effect of butyrate, discovered during a trial of the drug in 2002, was improved healing of the leg ulcers associated with sickle cell disease. This discovery led to a separate study in which twenty-five patients with a total of thirty-seven leg ulcers were given arginine butyrate. Several of these patients had struggled with leg ulcers for many years. Within three months, the average size of the ulcers had decreased by

53 percent. Seventeen of the ulcers were completely healed. Researchers continue to study arginine butyrate and its benefits to sickle cell patients.

Drugs to Improve Blood Flow

Other drugs with different beneficial effects are also being studied. Because acute pain episodes and severe crises are caused by the blockage of blood vessels when red blood cells become sickled, several therapies are being developed with the goal of preventing the causes of sickling, returning sickled cells to their normal shape, and improving the flow of cells through the vessels.

Nitric oxide is not actually a drug but is a gas that can meet several of these therapeutic goals. It is produced by special cells that line the walls of blood vessels. When inhaled, it is transported from the lungs by hemoglobin. Nitric oxide helps relax the walls of blood vessels and causes them to dilate, or become larger. This improves blood flow by itself, but nitric oxide can also prevent sickling of red cells and can actually "unsickle" sickled cells by melting the polymerized hemoglobin. "Hemoglobin S plus nitric oxide behaves much like normal adult hemoglobin," says one researcher. "This is not a cure, but we think it will get patients out of a crisis earlier or maybe prevent a crisis."[26] The use of nitric oxide to treat and shorten pain episodes is currently being studied at several research centers.

Dehydration of red cells is a well-known cause of sickling. In the early 1990s, researchers at Children's Hospital Boston discovered that a commonly used antifungal drug called clotrimazole helped to prevent red cells from losing water. Because the drug has some unpleasant potential side effects, researchers are working on other variations of the drug to find one that prevents sickling without the side effects.

Flocor is a relatively new drug that has been shown to decrease the length of pain episodes. In 2001, it was put on the development "fast track" by the FDA because of its apparent benefit to patients experiencing acute chest syndrome. Given intravenously, Flocor improves blood flow and oxygen delivery by putting a coating on damaged cells and on vessel walls, allowing the cells to slip over one another and through small blood vessels. It also changes the membranes of both normal and sickled cells, making them more flexible.

A Drug with Good Taste

The popular food flavoring vanilla may have a place in sickle cell treatment. Scientists have known for several decades that vanillin, the chemical that gives the vanilla bean its flavor, protects red cells from sickling. The effect had only been observed in the laboratory, however, because it could not be given by mouth. "If you give vanillin or vanilla to patients with sickle cell disease," explains one researcher, "all vanillin is destroyed in the stomach, because we have enzymes to destroy vanillin."[27]

The vanilla bean contains a chemical that looks promising for the treatment of sickle cell.

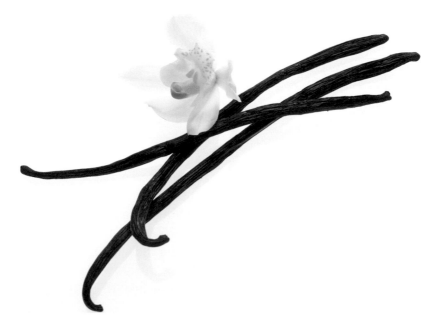

In 2004, a group of scientists in Philadelphia tested a variation of vanillin called MX-1520. MX-1520 is a prodrug, meaning that it turns into vanillin in the body. The scientists gave the MX-1520 to transgenic mice—mice that had been specially bred with the sickle cell gene. When exposed to low oxygen conditions, these mice developed a form of acute chest syndrome. The scientists found that when the mice were given MX-1520 before exposure to low oxygen, the percentage of sickle cells in the blood was significantly reduced, the crisis was avoided, and the mice lived much longer.

In addition to developing and improving treatment with medicines, other therapies are also being continually improved. Blood transfusion therapy, stem cell transplants, and gene therapy are all areas of great interest.

Predicting Strokes

In some sickle cell children, changes occur in the blood vessels of the brain that cause them to become narrow, making them more likely to become clogged with sickled cells and cause an ischemic stroke. Blood transfusions are effective at preventing strokes in children with sickle cell because they increase the percentage of healthy hemoglobin in the blood. Because of the possible complications associated with transfusions, however, it is always advisable to limit as much as possible the number of transfusions a child gets. A device called a transcranial Doppler (TCD) ultrasound can help with this.

The TCD ultrasound uses a handheld probe that sends out high-frequency sound waves that bounce off solid objects, such as blood vessels, and then turns the reflected sound waves into an image that can be viewed on a video screen. The ultrasound can show how narrow a blood vessel is. It can also measure the speed and quality of blood flow through the vessels. Higher speeds indicate a narrow passage and a potential site for a stroke. This allows doctors to identify which children are at a high risk for stroke and which are not and to limit frequent blood transfusions for those children who are found to be at high risk.

An Alternative Therapy for Strokes

Children who have had a stroke are at a very high risk of having more strokes. Regular blood transfusions help prevent them from happening, but doctors wanted to find an alternative to blood transfusions that would help prevent secondary strokes and, at the same time, reduce the hazards of iron overload. The nightly infusions of the chelating agent are difficult to tolerate for many patients, especially small children, and it can be difficult to persuade parents and their children to stay with the

Artificial Blood

Many symptoms and complications of sickle cell can be prevented or treated with blood transfusions. There are risks, however, associated with frequent transfusions, such as fluid and iron overload, disease transmission, and transfusion reactions.

Interest in the development of a safe and effective substitute for human blood began during World War II, for use on the battlefields. Such a product would also be useful for surgical patients, in disaster situations, and for accident victims who need blood replacement quickly but do not have time to wait for compatible blood. Interest intensified in the 1980s with the onset of the AIDS epidemic.

Several companies are currently working to develop blood substitutes that would be able to deliver oxygen safely without any dangerous side effects. Currently there are two different types being perfected. One is a red-colored product made from human or animal hemoglobin. The other is a purely artificial substance made from perfluorocarbons, or PFCs, a material similar to the non-stick coating Teflon. Liquid PFCs can carry a great deal of dissolved oxygen, about fifty times more than natural blood. This type of blood substitute has already been successfully used to treat severe acute chest syndrome.

therapy. It is also frequently unsuccessful at adequately relieving the iron overload. Two new developments offer improvements to transfusion and standard chelation therapy.

In November 2005, the FDA approved a new drug for treating transfusion-related iron overload called deferasirox. Instead of the difficult five-night-a-week infusion of the standard chelating agent, deferasirox is a tablet that can be taken once a day dissolved in liquid. This method of iron chelation is much easier for patients and families to comply with.

Most researchers today consider these products to be a companion treatment with blood rather than an absolute substitute; they do not replace all the functions of blood. Says Dr. Bruce Spiess of Virginia Commonwealth University, "I realized very early on that going head to head with a unit of blood was going to be very difficult. Instead ... go find some diseased states to treat that, right now, we don't have treatment for. If we can get it through the FDA, then we can use it in so many different ways. To treat stroke, for instance, or heart attacks, sickle cell anemia—even spinal cord injuries."

Quoted in Nicole Davis, "Better than Blood?" reprinted from Popular Science, November 2006. www.popsci.com/popsci/science/9e367f36fca9e010vgnvcm100004eecbccdrcrd.html.

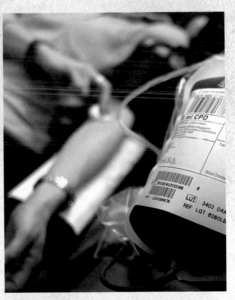

Artificial blood is being investigated for use in emergency transfusions such as accidents and severe acute chest syndrome.

A new study called the SWiTCH study is testing a different therapy for preventing second strokes and managing iron overload. It will compare the usual therapy of transfusion and chelation with a new method that combines the medication hydroxyurea with phlebotomy. Phlebotomy is a procedure in which blood is withdrawn from the patient in small amounts over time. The study will determine, first, if hydroxyurea is effective at preventing strokes and, second, if phlebotomy is effective for managing iron overload. If the new therapy is successful, it could dramatically decrease the number of blood transfusions a sickle cell patient gets.

Finding a Cure

New medications and improved treatment methods are providing longer and more comfortable lives for sickle cell patients, but the ultimate goal is still a cure, one that is available for all patients. Currently, stem cell transplant offers the only hope of a cure for sickle cell patients. Since the early years of bone marrow stem cell transplants, much has been learned about this revolutionary treatment and, to date, several hundred children have been cured of sickle cell with this procedure. Its success rate is close to 90 percent, and it is no longer considered experimental. It does have several important limitations, however, that reduce its availability to many patients. First, only about 10 to 25 percent of patients have a sibling who is a matched donor. Second, there is the risk that the patient's immune system will reject the donor stem cells and the transplant will not work. Third, there is the risk of graft-versus-host disease, a complication in which the donor tissue actually attacks the patient's cells. Fortunately, several advances have made these complications less likely. Alternative sources of stem cells and gene therapy are two possibilities that offer hope to many more patients for a final cure.

Haploidentical Transplants

Scientists at sickle cell treatment centers are researching ways to use donated cells from other family members, such as parents or siblings, who are not an exact tissue match to the patient. This is called a haploidentical transplant. Haploidentical transplants have been done successfully in patients with cancer and several kinds of noncancerous diseases. Because the donor marrow is not an exact match, it is processed in a special machine that separates out the stem cells from other marrow cells called T cells, which are known to trigger the rejection response, so that the chances of graft failure or GVIID are minimized. "A transplant is the only cure that's available to for children with sickle cell disease," says one scientist at St. Jude's Children's Research Hospital:

> but not many of our patients have a suitable match. In an attempt to provide this opportunity to more families, we need to find a different donor. Nearly everyone has a parent who's available, even if they don't have matched brothers or sisters. Haploidentical stem cell transplantation provides that curative option, so we're very excited about it.[28]

Stem Cells from Cord Blood

Bone marrow is only one source of stem cells. They can also be found in cord blood—the blood that remains inside the umbilical cord after a baby is born. Since the first cord blood transplant in 1988, over ten thousand of these transplants have been done worldwide. In 1998, Keone Penn, a young patient from Atlanta, Georgia, became the first sickle cell child to receive a transfusion of stem cells from cord blood. A year after Keone's transplant, his doctors declared him officially cured of sickle cell disease.

Cord blood stem cells may come from a newborn sibling or from an unrelated donor. They have certain advantages over bone marrow stem cells. They are more versatile because they come from a newborn infant whose immune system is not yet fully developed. For this reason, they are less likely to be rejected or cause GVHD, so they do not have to be as close a match to the patient as stem cells from older children or adults. Cord blood transplants are especially helpful for children because, although cord blood contains fewer stem cells, children do not need to receive as many as adults in order for the transplant to succeed.

Many children have been cured of sickle cell disease by the transfusion of stem cells from cord blood.

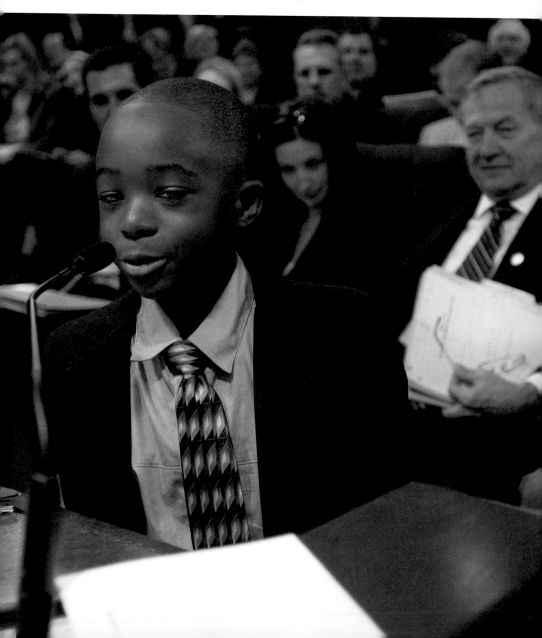

After years of trying to have a baby, the Davises' son Joseph was born. Then he was diagnosed with sickle cell disease. His symptoms were severe. "He wasn't even walking because of the pain," says his mother. His father adds, "He was just very sick all the time and unless we got a stem cell match, we didn't expect to have him very long."[29] After searching for a match for a year, the Davises were beginning to lose hope. Then, Mrs. Davis became pregnant with their son Isaac. Isaac turned out to be a good match for Joseph. Within months, Joseph received a transplant of stem cells from Isaac's cord blood. Their doctor explains, "[We] went in and collected the cord blood, provided those stem cells for transplant, and now the older child is cured of that disease."[30]

Cord blood can also be collected from the umbilical cords of newborns who are diagnosed with sickle cell disease before they are born and then used to treat the same child later. If pre-natal genetic tests have shown that a baby will have sickle cell disease, some of its cord blood can be collected at the time of his birth, frozen, and stored for future treatment of the child. Because the stem cells in the cord blood are the infant's own cells, there is no risk of tissue rejection or GVHD.

Researchers are currently working on ways to extract more stem cells from cord blood so that it will be even more effective in children and more useful in older patients as well. They are also looking at the effectiveness of combining stem cells from more than one donor in order to provide more cells during a transfusion. Meanwhile, knowledge about stem cell transplantation continues to grow. Scientists are finding that stem cell transplants can succeed even if only part of the patient's hemoglobin is converted to normal. This combination of healthy and unhealthy hemoglobin is called stable mixed chimerism. Both kinds of hemoglobin are present, but the healthy hemoglobin functions more effectively than the unhealthy hemoglobin, and the patient remains symptom-free. If this is true, then it may not be necessary to completely destroy patients' bone marrow with toxic drugs (myeloablation) before they receive a transplant. This non-myeloablative procedure would be much safer, with

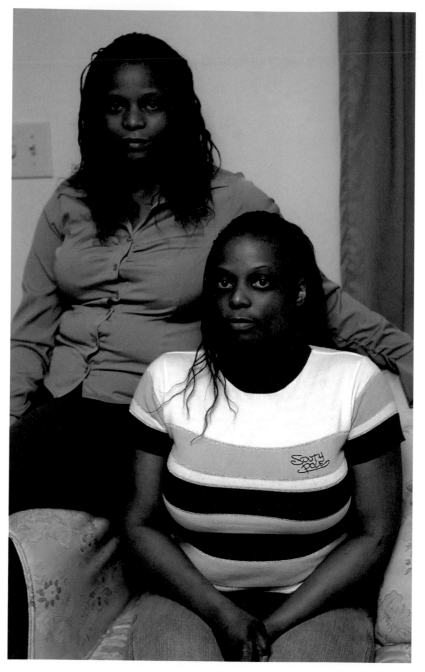

Children are living longer and more comfortable lives now because of improved screening and therapies.

less risk of toxicity from the drugs that are used. It would also preserve at least some of the patient's immune system. Doctors are very optimistic about this discovery. "The new protocol is let's go ahead and aim for the mixture so that it will allow transplants to be open to more people," explained Dr. Lewis Hsu, a pediatric sickle cell specialist at Emory University School of Medicine in Atlanta. "This could be the start of a very big step in the treatment of the disease."[31]

Gene Therapy for Sickle Cell Disease

Stem cell research holds a great deal of hope for a cure for sickle cell patients. Another area of research that holds promise is gene therapy—actually changing an individual's genetics to cure the disease. In 2001, scientists for the first time used specially-bred mice to correct sickle cell disease using gene therapy. The mice had been "bioengineered" to contain a human gene for sickle cell disease. Marrow from the sickle cell mice was removed and the stem cells genetically "corrected" by adding an antisickling gene. The new gene, called a transgene, produced a version of normal hemoglobin that does not sickle. The corrected cells were then transplanted into other mice whose own bone marrow had been destroyed by radiation. Three months later, the transplanted mice had a high level of the new, nonsickling hemoglobin in their blood. The mice also had many fewer irreversibly sickled cells in their blood. Two other signs of sickle cell, enlarged spleens and poorly concentrated urine, were also corrected with the new marrow.

In 2006, researchers at Memorial Sloan-Kettering Hospital in New York City used a new gene therapy strategy that also uses corrected transgenes to create normal hemoglobin. But these special transgenes had two jobs. They not only made normal hemoglobin, they could also stop any more abnormal hemoglobin S from being made. The new strategy is called RNA interference. RNA, or ribonucleic acid, is a close chemical relative of DNA, deoxyribonucleic acid. It has the ability to control how DNA expresses itself. In other words, if

DNA is the message, RNA is the messenger that carries the message to the part of the cell that makes the hemoglobin. In RNA interference, RNA is used to interfere with DNA's message to make Hb S. This new strategy is exciting because it offers hope for a cure without the obstacle of finding a matching stem cell donor. Instead, the cells come from the patients themselves.

The use of gene therapy to cure sickle cell disease is still very experimental, and a practical, safe, and effective way to apply it is still years in the future. The greatest obstacle at this point is ensuring that corrected genes are able to "express" themselves at a high enough level to make a difference. But interest in gene therapy is intense, and progress is being made.

How Do They Do It?

One of the greatest obstacles for gene therapy researchers to overcome is how to get new, corrected genes into enough cells to make a difference. Interestingly, the answer may lie with one of the most feared organisms in the world today—the Human Immunodeficiency Virus, the virus that causes AIDS.

Viruses are very tiny, submicroscopic particles that have their own DNA but are unable to reproduce themselves. They are very good, however, at injecting their DNA into the cells of a "host" organism, such as a person. They cause disease by invading healthy cells and using them to reproduce. Eventually, the cell contains so many viruses that it breaks open, allowing the viruses in it to spread to other host cells and start reproducing again.

The scientists who cured sickle cell disease in mice used a modified form of HIV to carry the corrected hemoglobin gene into the mice's red blood cells. This modified version cannot replicate itself inside the host cell, nor can it cause disease.

The next step in gene therapy will be to determine how safe it is to use the HIV vector in larger animals, specifically humans, and how safe it is when it is produced in large quantities.

A Reason for Optimism

Thirty years ago, only half of all children born with sickle cell disease lived to adulthood. Today, thanks to newborn screening, earlier treatment, improved medical therapies, and improved techniques for blood transfusion and stem cell transplant, the majority of sickle cell patients can look forward to longer and more comfortable lives. It may be only a matter of time before a safe and effective cure is available for this very complex disease.

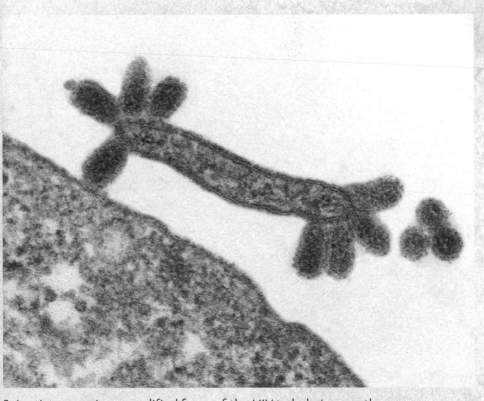

Scientists are using a modified form of the HIV to help in gene therapy.

Notes

Introduction: An Old Disease with a New Name

1. Miriam Bloom, PhD, *Understanding Sickle Cell Disease.* Jackson, MS: University Press of Mississippi, 1995, p. 24.
2. Bloom, p. 24.
3. Alan F. Platt Jr., PA-C, and Alan Sacerdote, MD, *Hope and Destiny.* Roscoe, IL: Hilton Publishing Co., 2002, p. 131.

Chapter One: What Is Sickle Cell Disease?

4. Quoted in "Sickle Cell Anemia," Iron Disorders Institute, 2006. www.irondisorders.org/Disorders/Sickle-Cell.asp
5. Bloom, p. 41.
6. Quoted in "Housing Project Works to Help Sickle Cell Patients," NPR broadcast of the Tavis Smiley Show, September 29, 2004. www.npr.org/templates/story/story. php?storyID=4052529.

Chapter Two: Symptoms and Complications

7. Quoted in Alan and Virginia Silverstein and Laura Silverstein Nunn, *Sickle Cell Anemia.* Springfield, NJ: Enslow Publishers, Inc., 1997, p. 56.
8. Quoted in "Patients' Stories: Real Life Testimonies for Help and Inspiration," The Sickle Cell Information Center, 1997. www.scinfo.org/ptstory.htm.
9. Silverstein and Nunn, p. 31.
10. Platt and Sacerdote, p. 156.
11. Silverstein and Nunn, p. 34.

Chapter Three: Diagnosis and Treatment

12. Quoted in Toni Baker, "Like a New Life," *MCG Today,* Medical College of Georgia, Spring, 2006, Vol. 33, No. 4. www.mcg.edu/News/MCGToday/Spr06/Story4.htm.

13. Quoted in "Serious Illness Among Children with Sickle Cell Disease Reduced with Vaccine," *Science Daily*, May 4, 2007. www.sciencedaily.com/releases/2007/05/070501115006.htm.

14. Quoted in David Williamson, "Major Study: Hydroxyurea Reduces Sickle Cell Mortality by 40 Percent," News release from University of North Carolina, April 1, 2003. www.unc.edu/news/archives/apr03/orringer040103.html.

15. Quoted in "Lloyd's Video Diary," Great Ormond Street Hospital for Children, London. Courtesy of CBBC Newsround, November 23, 2006. www.childrenfirst.nhs.uk/teens/gosh_tv/lloyd/index.html.

16. Quoted in Toni Baker, "Ironing Out the Problem," *MCG Today*, Medical College of Georgia, Spring, 2006, Vol. 33, No. 4. www.mcg.edu/News/MCGToday/Spr06/Story2.htm.

17. Quoted in "Bone Marrow Transplant for Sickle Cell Disease," Children's Hospital of Pittsburgh, 2007. www.chp.edu/centers/03trans_success_jones.php.

18. Quoted in "Bone Marrow Transplant for Sickle Cell Disease."

Chapter Four: Living with Sickle Cell Disease

19. Quoted in "Sickle Cell Sufferers Living Longer, Dying Less from Their Disease," News release from University of Texas Southwestern Medial Center, March 25, 2004. www.utsouthwestern.edu/utsw/cda/dept37389/files/158834.html.

20. Quoted in "Sickle Cell Anemia," Iron Disorders Institute, 2006. www.irondisorders.org/Disorders/Sickle-Cell.asp.

21. Quoted in "Living with Sickle Cell Anemia," BBC News, May 1, 2007. http://news.bbc.co.uk/2/hi/africa/6646289.stm.

22. "Lloyd's Video Diary."

Chapter Five: On the Horizon

23. Quoted in "Hope for Babies with Sickle Cell Disease," *Promise* Magazine, Spring, 2006. St. Jude's Children's Research Hospital. www.stjude.org/media/0,2561,453_5716_20750,00.html.

24. Quoted in Baker, "Like a New Life."
25. Quoted in "Vanilla May Have a Future in Sickle Cell Treatment," *Science Daily*, September 21, 2004. www. sciencedaily.com/releases/2004/09/040921075701.htm.
26. Quoted in Toni Baker, "Inhaled Nitric Oxide May Help Sickle Cell Disease," *MCG News*, Medical College of Georgia, October 21, 2005. https://my.mcg.edu/portal/page/portal/News/archive/2005/Inhaled%20nitric%20oxide%20may%20help%20sickle%20cell%20disease.
27. Quoted in Bob Hirshon, "Vanilla Medicine," Transcript of Science NetLinks audio file, 2006. www.sciencenetlinks.com/sci_update.cfm?DocID=238.
28. Quoted in "Two More Miracles," *Promise* Magazine, St. Jude's Children's Research Hospital, Winter, 2006. www.stjude.org/feature/0,2703,616_5496_19960,00.html.
29. Quoted in Suleika Acosta, "New Arizona Law Could Save Lives," KOLD News, Tucson, AZ, January 21, 2007. www.kold.com/Global/story.asp?S=5916984.
30. Acosta, "New Arizona Law Could Save Lives."
31. Quoted in Patricia Guthrie, "Gentler Treatment for Sickle Cell Hailed," *Atlanta Journal Constitution*, October 26, 2001. www.stopsicklecell.com/news2.asp.

Glossary

acidosis: Abnormally high acid level in the blood and body tissues.

acute chest syndrome: A very serious complication of sickle cell disease, caused by a sickling episode in the lungs, with symptoms similar to severe pneumonia.

alloimmunization: A reaction to frequent blood transfusions in which the immune system begins to attack compatible donated blood as if it were not compatible.

amino acids: The small chemical units that make up the structure of proteins.

amniocentesis: A diagnostic test in which amniotic fluid is withdrawn from the uterus during pregnancy and the cells in it are examined for genetic abnormalities.

anemia: A condition of the blood in which there are not enough healthy red cells, or enough healthy hemoglobin in them, to provide adequate oxygen to the tissues.

antibiotics: Medications that prevent or treat infections caused by bacteria. They are not effective against viruses.

antibodies: Proteins on the surface of immune system cells that neutralize foreign particles such as bacteria, viruses, parasites, or donated tissues by binding specifically to them.

aplastic crisis: A serious and painful complication of sickle cell disease in which an infarction in the bones causes the marrow to completely stop producing red cells.

apoplexy: The old term for stroke, coined by the ancient Greeks.

auto-splenectomy: A phenomenon in which the spleen, after repeated damage from sickle cell disease, shrinks and eventually disappears.

bilirubin: A by-product of red cell destruction that serves a function in digestion of fatty foods.

blood transfusion: The administration of blood from a donor into the bloodstream of a patient.

carbon dioxide: A gaseous waste product of metabolism that is removed from the body in exhalation from the lungs.

cardiologist: A doctor who specializes in diseases and disorders of the heart and blood vessels.

chelating agent: A medication that helps the body excrete excess iron in the blood.

chelation: The process of administering a chelating agent to rid the body of excess iron.

chimerism: A balance of genetically different tissue in the same organism. In sickle cell disease, it refers to a balance of both abnormal hemoglobin and normal hemoglobin made by donated stem cells.

chorionic villus sampling: A diagnostic test in which a small piece of chorionic villi is removed during pregnancy and tested for genetic abnormalities.

chromosomes: Threadlike structures found in the cell nucleus that contain the genes.

chronic: Long-term, lasting for months or years.

complete blood count (CBC): A blood test that measures the amounts and characteristics of the various cells in the blood. Used most often for detecting infection or anemia.

creatinine: A metabolic by-product whose measurement helps indicate kidney function.

DNA: Deoxyribonucleic acid, the chemical substance that genes are made of.

dominant trait: A genetic trait that shows if even only one gene for the trait has been inherited.

electrophoresis: A chemical method of separating and measuring different types of proteins according to their response to an electric field.

erythrocytes: The medical term for red blood cells.

erythropoietin: A type of growth hormone that stimulates the bone marrow to produce red cells.

fetal hemoglobin: The kind of hemoglobin that infants are born with. It protects against sickling but is replaced by adult hemoglobin by about six months of age.

folic acid: A B vitamin that supports the manufacture of red cells by the bone marrow.

gallstones: Small stones, made from the build-up in the gallbladder of substances such as bile, salts, cholesterol, and bilirubin, which can block the ducts leading out of the gallbladder and cause disease.

gene: A unit of DNA, located on a chromosome, that carries the code or a specific characteristic.

genetic: Any characteristic that is inherited from one's parents.

glutamic acid: The amino acid in the beta chain of hemoglobin that is replaced by another amino acid called valine, which causes sickle cell disease.

graft-versus-host disease: A condition in which donated tissue attacks the patient's tissues as if they were the foreign substance.

HLA system: Human Leukocyte Antigen system, for identifying antigens on tissue cells to find tissue matches between donors and recipients.

hand-foot syndrome: An early sign of sickle cell disease, seen in infants and small children, in which sickling causes painful swelling of the hands and feet.

haploidentical: A term referring to tissue such as stem cells that are donated by a family member who is a close, but not exact, tissue match to the patient.

hematocrit: A measurement of the percentage of volume in the blood taken up by the red cells. Normal hematocrit varies by age but ranges from 42 percent to 64 percent for newborns and 36 percent to 49 percent for teens.

hematologist: A doctor who specializes in diagnosing and treating blood disorders.

hematuria: The medical term for blood in the urine. Can indicate kidney disease or infection.

hemoglobin: The protein in red cells that gives blood its red color and binds to oxygen.

hemoglobin beta gene: The gene that carries the genetic instructions for making hemoglobin.

hemolysis: The term for the destruction or breakage of red blood cells.

hydroxyurea: A cancer treatment drug that has been shown to be effective in preventing sickling by stimulating production of fetal hemoglobin.

infarction: The blockage of blood flow and oxygen supply to the tissue cells, causing tissue death.

intracerebral hemorrhage: A kind of stroke in which a blood vessel in the brain ruptures and causes bleeding in the brain.

in vitro fertilization: A procedure in which egg cells are fertilized by sperm cells outside the body and then implanted into the mother's womb.

ischemic stroke: A kind of stroke in which a blood vessel in the brain is obstructed and oxygen cannot get to the tissue.

jaundice: The yellowish discoloration of the skin and eyes caused by build-up of bilirubin in the blood. Usually indicates liver disease.

malaria: A serious, tropical disease that appears in milder form in people with sickle cell trait.

marrow: The dark, spongy material inside the larger bones that produces stem cells.

meningitis: An inflammation of the tissue surrounding the brain and spinal cord.

metabolism: The chemical processes that take place in the body's cells that allow them to grow, reproduce, and carry out their particular functions.

mutation: A genetic mistake in a gene that causes faulty information to be given to the cells, causing disease or deformity.

myeloablation: The process of temporarily destroying a person's bone marrow so that his or her natural immunity will not cause rejection of transplanted tissue.

necrosis: Tissue breakdown, usually caused by an inadequate oxygen supply.

nucleus: The structure in the center of most cells that contains all the genetic information in the chromosomes.

oxygen: A gas that makes up 21 percent of the air and is necessary for life.

pH: A measurement of the acidity of a fluid. Neutral pH is 7.0;

the lower the pH, the more acidic the fluid. Normal blood pH is between 7.35 and 7.45.

parasite: An organism that lives on or in another organism and may cause it harm. The organism that causes malaria is a parasite.

persistent fetal hemoglobin: A mutation that permits a person to produce fetal hemoglobin much longer than normal, even into adulthood.

phagocytes: Immune system cells that attack and destroy foreign particles such as bacteria, viruses, and parasites.

phlebotomy: The technique of drawing blood out of a vein with a needle and syringe.

pneumococcal conjugate vaccine (PCV): The vaccine that prevents people from getting infections caused by the pneumococcus bacterium.

pneumonia: An infection of the lungs that causes fluid build-up, difficulty breathing, and fever.

polymers: Rod-like structures made of abnormal hemoglobin that cause red cells to become sickle-shaped and sticky.

preimplantation genetic diagnosis: A procedure in which, after egg cells are fertilized in vitro, they are tested for genetic disease, and only the healthy embryos are implanted in the mother.

proteins: Large organic compounds made up of chains of amino acids, the sequence of which is genetically determined. Proteins are part of all living organisms and participate in every cell function.

RNA: Ribonucleic acid. Closely related chemically to DNA, RNA translates the DNA instructions for making proteins.

recessive trait: A trait that requires inheritance of both genes from the parents in order for the characteristic to show in the individual.

red blood cells: Cells in the blood that contain hemoglobin and carry oxygen to all other cells in the body.

septicemia: An infection of the blood.

sickle-beta thalassemia: A variation of sickle cell anemia in which a child inherits one gene for sickle cell disease and one gene for beta thalassemia.

sickle cell crisis: An episode of pain, often severe, caused by sickled cells obstructing blood flow to a particular part of the body.

sickle cell trait: The condition in which a person has inherited one sickle cell gene and one normal gene.

splenectomy: Surgical removal of the spleen.

splenic sequestration: A type of crisis in which a large number of red cells become trapped in the spleen, causing intense pain, swelling of the spleen, and severe anemia.

stem cells: Cells made in the bone marrow that have not yet specialized into any particular type of cell.

stroke: An event that takes place in the brain in which a portion of the brain tissue becomes deprived of its oxygen supply.

thalassemia: A group of related blood disorders that cause inadequate amounts of hemoglobin and varying degrees of anemia.

transcranial Doppler ultrasound: A diagnostic procedure in which high-frequency sound waves are reflected off structures in the head and turned into an image of the structures.

transfusion reaction: An immune response, similar to an allergic reaction, in which the immune system of a person receiving a blood transfusion attacks the donated blood.

transgene: A gene that has been transferred by genetic engineering techniques from one organism to another.

vaccine: A medication made from microorganisms that have been killed or made harmless that, when administered, protects a person from getting the disease normally caused by the microorganism.

valine: The amino acid that takes the place of glutamic acid in the hemoglobin chain and causes the body to make sickle cell hemoglobin.

Organizations to Contact

American Sickle Cell Anemia Association

Cleveland Clinic, East Office Building
10300 Carnegie Avenue
Cleveland, OH 44106
216-229-8600
www.ascaa.org
Executive Director Ira Bragg: irabragg@ascaa.org

Provides a wide range of services to people with sickle cell or related diseases, including testing, counseling, education, and support.

Iron Disorders Institute

2722 Wade Hampton Blvd, Suite A
Greenville, SC 29615
864-292 1175
www.irondisorders.org
PatientServices@ironisorders.org

IDI's purpose is to help people with iron disorders and other blood disorders receive an early and accurate diagnosis, get appropriate treatment, and live in good health.

National Heart, Lung, and Blood Institute

NHLBI Health Information Center
P.O. Box 30105
Bethesda, MD 20824-0105
301-592-8573
www.nhlbi.nih.gov
nhlbiinfo@nhlbi.nih.gov

The NHLBI plans, conducts, and supports basic research

and education projects with an emphasis on the causes, prevention, diagnosis, and treatment of heart, blood vessel, lung, and blood diseases and sleep disorders.

Sickle Cell Disease Association of America
231 E. Baltimore St., Suite 800
Baltimore, MD 21202
1-800-421-8453
www.sicklecelldisease.org
scdaa@sicklecelldisease.org

The mission of the SCDAA is to raise awareness of sickle cell disease, to provide education for patients and health professionals, to improve the quality of life for all patients, and to support research into finding a universal cure for sickle cell.

For More Information

Books

Carol Baldwin, *Sickle Cell Disease*. Chicago, IL: Heineman Library, 2003. A clearly written and well-illustrated overview of sickle cell disease designed for younger readers.

Miriam Bloom, PhD, *Understanding Sickle Cell Disease*. Jackson, MS: University Press of Mississippi, 1995. A very thorough overview of sickle cell disease. Lots of detail, but easy to understand.

Susan Dudley Gold, *Sickle Cell Disease*. Berkeley Heights, NJ: Enslow Publishers, Inc., 2001. The story of Keone Penn, the first sickle cell patient to receive a cord blood transplant.

Melanie Gordon, *Let's Talk About Sickle Cell Anemia*. New York: Power Kids Press, 2000. A simple introduction to a complex disease, good for young readers.

Allan F. Platt Jr., PA-C, and Alan Sacerdote, MD, *Hope and Destiny: A Patient's and Parent's Guide to Sickle Cell Disease and Sickle Cell Trait*. Roscoe, IL: Hilton Publishing Company, 2002. Informative guide for patients, families, and loved ones that covers the physical and emotional aspects of the disease through all stages of a patient's life.

Alvin and Virginia Silverstein and Laura Silverstein Nunn, *Sickle Cell Anemia*. Berkeley Heights, NJ: Enslow Publishers, Inc., 1997. A thorough and well-written explanation of sickle cell disease for middle school students.

Web Sites

About Sickle Cell (http://k12education.uams.edu/scvlab/about.htm). All about the disease, its history, biology of the blood, and how sickling occurs.

Information Center for Sickle Cell and Thalassemic Disorders (http://sickle.bwh.harvard.edu/). This site provides a source of current information on sickle cell disease, thalassemia, and disorders of iron metabolism.

KidsHealth (www.kidshealth.org). Presented by the Nemours foundation, provides health information on a variety of topics, including sickle cell disease, for parents, kids, and teens.

Sickle Cell Kids (www.SickleCellKids.org). Colorful, interactive, kid-friendly site with games, stories, and letters from celebrities.

Sickle Cell Information Center (www.scinfo.org). Provides sickle cell patients, families, and health professionals with information, education, news, research updates, and links to worldwide sickle cell resources.

The Sickle Cell Information Center at Grady Health System (www.scinfo.org). Provides the sickle cell patient and professional with education, news, research updates, and worldwide sickle cell resources.

Index

Picture Credits

Cover, © Lester V. Bergman/Corbis
Alfred Pasieka/Photo Researchers, Inc., 43
AP Images, 17, 19, 25, 34, 40, 45, 61, 86, 88
Astrid Kage/Photo Researchers, Inc., 30
Beth Galton/FoodPix/Jupiter Images, 47
© Bettmann/Corbis, 11, 35, 49
Brian Hagiwara/Brand X Pictures/Jupiter Images, 47
Brian Hagiwara/FoodPix/Jupiter Images, 47
Burke/Triolo Productions/FoodPix/Jupiter Images, 80
Comstock Images/Jupiter Images, 7
Created by Avila Creative Design, 12, 13, 15, 59, 77
Dr. P. Marazzi/Photo Researchers, Inc., 27
Faye Norman/Photo Researchers, Inc., 51
© Image Source/Corbis, 65
© Jim Craigmyle/Corbis, 73
Maximilian Stock Ltd./FoodPix/Jupiter Images, 47
Michelle Del Guercio/Photo Researchers, Inc., 42
© moodboard/Corbis, 69
© Richard Eric Henderson/Corbis, 66
© Sean Justice/Corbis, 71
© Sora/Corbis, 46
SPL/Photo Researchers, Inc., 56
Steve Gschmeissner / Photo Researchers, Inc., 91
Sue Ford/Photo Researchers, Inc., 37
© Toby Melville/Reuters/Corbis, 83
© Valentin Ogneov/COVER/Corbis, 19
VOISIN/Photo Researchers, Inc., 73

About the Author

Lizabeth Peak received her Bachelor of Science in Nursing from the University of Florida in 1978 and her Bachelor of Science in Secondary Education from Southwest Missouri State University in 1991. She currently works full time as a surgical nurse, specializing in general and vascular surgery.

Lizabeth has published both fiction and nonfiction works for both adults and children. She especially enjoys writing about history, biography, and medical topics. She lives in Springfield, Missouri, with her husband Brian, daughters Rebecca and Wendy, three dogs, and two cats. When she is not working or writing, she enjoys hiking, reading, and St. Louis Cardinals baseball.

"Sickle Cell Disease" is her second book for Lucent Books.